Cystitis - Updates and Challenges

Edited by Giovanni Palleschi and Antonio Cardi

Published in London, United Kingdom

Cystitis - Updates and Challenges
http://dx.doi.org/10.5772/intechopen.105317
Edited by Giovanni Palleschi and Antonio Cardi

Contributors
Skander Essafi, Maha Abid, Sana Rouis, Amel Omezzine Letaief, Dragana Živković, Maja Samardžić Lukić, Asad Ullah, Muhammad Jamil, Carlos Arturo Levi D'Ancona, André Canettieri Rubez, Seçkin Engin, Giovanni Palleschi

First published in London, United Kingdom, 2023 by IntechOpen
IntechOpen is the global imprint of INTECHOPEN LIMITED, registered in England and Wales, registration number: 11086078, 5 Princes Gate Court, London, SW7 2QJ, United Kingdom

British Library Cataloguing-in-Publication Data
A catalogue record for this book is available from the British Library

Additional hard and PDF copies can be obtained from orders@intechopen.com

Cystitis - Updates and Challenges
Edited by Giovanni Palleschi and Antonio Cardi
p. cm.
Print ISBN 978-1-83768-849-4
Online ISBN 978-1-83768-850-0
eBook (PDF) ISBN 978-1-83768-851-7

For EU product safety concerns:
IN TECH d.o.o., Prolaz Marije Krucifikse Kozulić 3, 51000 Rijeka, Croatia,
info@intechopen.com or visit our website at intechopen.com.

Meet the editors

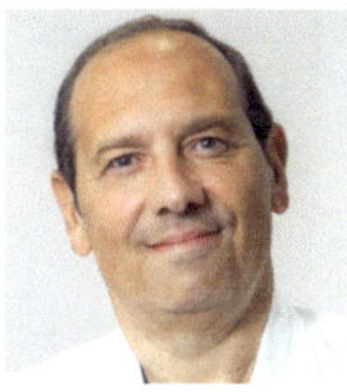

Giovanni Palleschi, MD, Ph.D., obtained an MD in Medicine and Surgery in 1997 and a specialization in Urology in 2002. He also obtained two master's degrees in Laparoscopy in 2005 and 2022, respectively, and a Ph.D. in Anatomy, Plastic Surgery and Dermatology in 2008. He previously taught courses in medicine and nursing. He is the author of seventy manuscripts and scientific books. He has been a speaker and organizer of numerous scientific events and a co-investigator in clinical trials. Dr. Palleschi is a previous board member of the Italian Society of Urodynamics (SIUD), the scientific committees of SIUD, the Italian Society of Urology (SIU), and the European Society of Urology (EAU), and several teaching committees. He is the winner of six scientific awards. He is a reviewer and editor for journals, including *Frontiers in Urology, Biology, Toxins, Diagnostics, and Biomedicine.* He is a member of the Italian Botulinum Toxin Network and a consultant for the Dialysis and Kidney Transplant Registry.

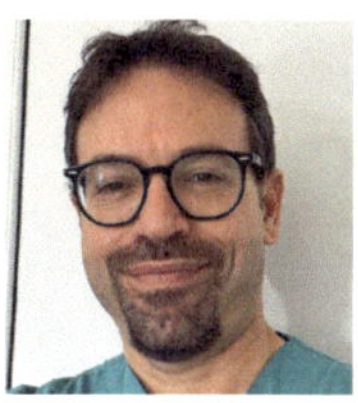

Antonio Cardi is a surgeon with a degree in medicine and surgery from the University of Rome "La Sapienza," Italy, where he graduated with a 110 cum laude distinction and was a winner of the Specialization Competition in Urology. Dr. Cardi obtained a specialization diploma in urology with honors, and his research activities include laparoscopic urological surgery. He holds a Ph.D. in New Technologies in Surgery and has been involved in numerous research activities, presenting abstracts at various congresses and conferences. Throughout his career, Dr. Cardi has worked in different hospitals and institutions, gaining valuable experience in laparoscopic surgeries, robotic surgery, and urological oncology. He currently works at the Urology Unit of San Giovanni Addolorata, Rome, Italy, specializing in robotic surgery and other advanced urological procedures. Dr. Cardi's contributions to the field have been remarkable, having performed more than 300 major robotic surgeries as the primary surgeon.

Contents

Preface **IX**

Prologue **XI**

Chapter 1 **1**
Introductory Chapter: Presenting an Overview on the Main Clinical, Diagnostic and Therapeutic Aspects of Human Cystitis
by Giovanni Palleschi

Chapter 2 **5**
Recurrent Cystitis in Women: Optimal Recommended Diagnostic Evaluation, Management and Prevention Options
by Skander Essafi, Maha Abid, Sana Rouis and Amel Omezzine Letaief

Chapter 3 **27**
Cystitis in Children
by Dragana Živković and Maja Samardžić Lukić

Chapter 4 **43**
Interstitial Cystitis/Bladder Pain Syndrome
by Asad Ullah and Muhammad Jamil

Chapter 5 **67**
Radiation Cystitis
by Carlos Arturo Levi D'Ancona and André Canettieri Rubez

Chapter 6 **83**
Drug-Related Cystitis: An Overview
by Seçkin Engin

Preface

Bladder inflammation is described as cystitis, a pathological condition caused by microbial agents and a common urinary tract infection (UTI). Although the prevalence of infectious cystitis is increasing worldwide, often representing a therapeutic challenge due to the resistance to antibiotics expressed by the responsible pathogens, bladder inflammation also recognizes different etiopathogenetic mechanisms. In fact, several non-infectious diseases may determine bladder inflammation, which is responsible for bothersome symptoms such as increased micturition frequency, urinary urgency, urinary burning, urinary incontinence, bladder pain, and hematuria. Various studies have shown that the impact of cystitis on a patient's quality of life is strongly negative, especially when the inflammation recurs or becomes chronic, causing pain or discomfort that is difficult to eradicate. The literature provides several data on various types of cystitis, however, most of these manuscripts focus only on a specific type of bladder inflammation, providing updates or describing results of research that explain new pathogenetic mechanisms or propose new therapeutic strategies. There is a lack of publications specifically dedicated to describing all main types of cystitis. As such, this book provides a comprehensive overview of the most important categories of cystitis. Written by experts in the field, this book includes six chapters.

Chapter 1: "Introductory Chapter: Presenting an Overview on the Main Clinical, Diagnostic and Therapeutic Aspects of Human Cystitis"

Chapter 2: "Recurrent Cystitis in Women: Optimal Recommended Diagnostic Evaluation, Management and Prevention Options"

Chapter 3: "Cystitis in Children"

Chapter 4: "Interstitial Cystitis/Bladder Pain Syndrome"

Chapter 5: "Radiation Cystitis"

Chapter 6: "Drug-Related Cystitis: An Overview"

After an introductory chapter that presents a general overview of the topic, the book moves on to a discussion of bacterial cystitis in adults. Today, there are several doubts about the correct approach to treat this condition, particularly recurrent bacterial cystitis, due to the abuse of antibiotics in the last years and the consequent increase of bacterial resistance to drugs expressed by the most common etiopathogenetic agents of *Escherichia coli, Klebsiella pneumoniae, Proteus mirabilis, Enterococcus faecalis,* and *Staphylococcus saprophyticus*. Chapter 2 provides evidence of the current etiopathogenetic aspects of bacterial cystitis, reviews proper diagnostic procedures, and discusses recommended treatment to limit bacterial resistance and thus prevent the recurrence of infection. The chapter also discusses the prevention of cystitis. Chapter 3 is dedicated to pediatric patients. Inappropriate management of infectious disease in pediatric patients may lead to severe complications that can become life-threatening or chronic. In addition, therapeutic regimens in childhood are different from those in adults. Chapter 4 discusses the diagnosis and therapeutic management of interstitial cystitis. Many patients with this condition, almost all of whom are women, receive a late diagnosis because the early clinical presentation of the disease is often misinterpreted as an infectious disease. Chapter 5 discusses radiation cystitis. Radiation therapy has become the standard treatment for many tumors, especially those involving the pelvic area. Despite the reduction of inflammatory complications by new devices, the number of patients undergoing radiation therapy is increasing and a significant number of these patients experience radiation cystitis. As the population ages, more patients are developing neoplastic conditions of the pelvic area. Elderly patients may not be eligible for surgery and thus they may need to undergo radiation therapy. Furthermore, this therapeutic option is very often used as adjuvant treatment after surgery of the prostate and bladder (and some other tumors of this anatomic area), and cystitis can be a frequent consequence. Finally, Chapter 6 examines drug-related cystitis. Some pharmacological agents used in chronic treatments can be the cause of severe bladder inflammation. Being that iatrogenic cystitis is rare, its diagnosis and treatment are not well-known by clinicians. An important aspect that must be considered is the cost of diagnosis and treatment of cystitis, as the prevalence of this condition is increasing worldwide. The expense of antibiotics constitutes a real economic emergency in healthcare systems and is partly due to inappropriate use of these drugs due to inadequate knowledge of guidelines and recommended therapeutic regimens.

This book presents diagnostic-therapeutic schemes useful in daily clinical practice for using effective therapies and preventing abuse of antibiotics and thus limiting the development of drug resistance. This aspect is particularly important because clinical research has not yet introduced new drugs onto the market that can overcome the limits caused by the resistance of microorganisms, which in some cases can cause severe clinical conditions for patients, especially those who are hospitalized or immunosuppressed. With reference to non-infectious cystitis, the therapeutic approach often takes little consideration of relevant guidelines because the treatment options are not always readily available. However, this can lead to an aggravation of the disease with a very negative impact on the patient's quality of life. Therefore, especially in non-infectious cystitis, which is discussed in this book, a medical intervention must strictly adhere to current guidelines in order to choose the appropriate therapies and limit chronicity and worsening of the disease to improve patient quality of life.

I want to thank all the contributing authors for their participation, effort, professionalism, and clinical and scientific expertise.

Giovanni Palleschi, MD, Urologist, Ph.D.
Hemodialysis Unit,
Nefrocenter Group,
Frascati, Rome, Italy

Antonio Cardi
San Giovanni Addolorato Hospital,
Urology Unit,
Rome, Italy

Prologue

Inflammatory disorders of the urinary tract have high incidence and prevalence worldwide. These conditions affect women and men from childhood to old age and therefore have a significant negative impact on quality of life, being sometimes responsible for severe, life-threatening complications. Cystitis is the most prevalent inflammatory condition of the urinary tract. It is responsible for bothering symptoms, but very often it is clinically underestimated for several reasons. Many patients have the habit of self-managing this condition when symptoms develop, using antibiotics and anti-inflammatory drugs without consulting a doctor or undergoing laboratory examinations or other diagnostic tests. This is very common, especially among women and it is one of the most important reasons for the significant increase of bacterial resistance to drugs in the last years as well as the high incidence of recurrent or chronic cystitis. There is also the common idea that cystitis could be only the consequence of bacterial infections; however, many inflammations of the bladder have a non-infectious origin, even if the symptoms are similar. Furthermore, non-infectious cystitis is usually chronic and difficult to treat, often representing a challenge for clinicians because its pathophysiologic mechanisms are still not completely understood and therapies in some cases are still experimental. This book reviews the different types of cystitis, providing detailed information on etiopathogenesis, pathophysiology, and treatments. It is an important guide for clinical practice not only for specialists but also for general practitioners. In addition, the text can also be consulted by patients, helping them to seek proper medical intervention instead of self-medicating.

Valeria Rossi
Nephrologist,
Chief of Nefrocenter Haemodialysis Centre,
Frascati, Rome, Italy

Chapter 1

Introductory Chapter: Presenting an Overview on the Main Clinical, Diagnostic and Therapeutic Aspects of Human Cystitis

Giovanni Palleschi

1. Introduction

Bladder inflammation is identified as cystitis. Among the different classification systems of urinary tract infections (UTIs), cystitis represents the most prevalent condition. Bladder inflammation does not recognize infections as the only etiopathogenetic factor. In fact, several non infectious diseases may determine bladder inflammation and are often chronic. In both cases, cystitis is responsible for highly bothering symptoms: increase of micturition frequency, urinary urgency (the complaint of a sudden compelling desire to pass urine that is difficult to defer), urinary burning, urinary incontinence, bladder pain/discomfort, and hematuria, rarely associated with fever. All these symptoms have a negative impact on patients' quality of life because especially in some conditions they recur or persist for a long time [1]. Uncomplicated cystitis are those acute, sporadic, or recurrent cystitis with no known relevant anatomical and functional abnormalities with the urinary tract or significant associated comorbidities [2]. Usually microbial cystitis in men are not common because almost in all cases there is an associated inflammation of the prostate (prostatitis). Therefore, when symptoms of UTIs develop in men and the treatment needs antimicrobials, drugs penetrating the prostatic tissue are recommended. Complicated cases are those in whom some clinical features of the patient (comorbidities, anatomical abnormalities) can determine a condition that is more difficult to treat: diabetes, congenital anatomic disorders, and state of immunosuppression are the most represented factors increasing the risk of complications. However, both men and women can be affected by abacterial cystitis that include various clinical conditions and recognize etherogeneous etiopathogenetic agents.

2. Background from literature

Current literature provides data on various types of cystitis. However, most of the manuscripts focus the attention on a single, specific subtype of cystitis and a large amount of data are available especially about interstitial cystitis, and chronic bladder pain (bladder pain syndrome). In the last years, poor data have been published on bacterial cystitis, as on radiation cystitis, or cystitis related to drugs. A very important

IntechOpen

topic is the bacterial resistance to antimicrobial drugs that is becoming even more critical especially in hospitalized individuals. Therefore, the recent literature lacks a text that summarizes the most significant topics about cystitis and can represent a sort of guide for clinical practice.

3. Main topics in the field of cystitis

There are some main topics that need to be discussed about cystitis. Nowadays, bacterial cystitis have become difficult to treat due to the abuse of antibiotics in the last years that caused a significant increase of germs' resistance to drugs the abuse of antibiotics in the last 10 years and the consequent increase of bacterial resistance to drugs. Therefore, it is important to provide an update on the current etiopathogenetic aspects of bacterial cystitis, and especially to focus the attention on the correct diagnostic procedures and the recommended treatment which aims to limit the bacterial resistance preventing the recurrence of the infection. In fact, the prevention of cystitis is also an underconsidered topic and poor data are available from literature regarding lifestyle changes that can reduce the onset of this condition and limit the recurrence rate [3]. Bladder pain syndrome is a very discussed argument and includes various conditions that still represent a challenge for clinicians. In particular, still today diagnostic and therapeutic management of Interstitial Cystitis is under debate and therefore continuous update is required for urologists and gynecologists, considering the hard negative impact that this condition causes on patients [4]. Radiation therapy has become the standard treatment for many tumors, especially those involving the pelvic area. Despite the incidence of inflammatory complications that has been reduced by new devices available for this treatment, the number of patients undergoing radiation therapy is increasing during the time and a significant group of subjects experience radiation cystitis [5]. While in many cases the inflammation is mild and easily managed in primary care, sometimes it could be severely bothering and responsible for complications that can become a risk for life. Another type of iatrogenic cystitis can be the consequence of the administration of specific drugs. Some pharmacological agents used in chronic treatments can be the cause of severe bladder inflammation. Being this condition not very frequent, its diagnosis, and especially its treatment, are not well known by clinicians. Urinary tract infections can be frequent in immunocompromised patients or in subjects that still need to develop a complete immunological competence. That is the case of pediatric subjects, who need specific assessment and dedicated diagnostic and therapeutic algorithm, considering also the fact that symptoms sometimes can be deceiving.

4. Considerations about real clinical practice

One of the most important challenges nowadays in this field, specifically regarding real clinical practice, is therefore to prevent the recurrence of bacterial cystitis, to improve the efficacy of antimicrobial agents against multiresistant bacteria, to reduce the risk of chronicization, and to find more effective therapeutic strategies to fight abacterial cystitis. When cystitis becomes very frequent, with high recurrence, or takes on a chronic course, it causes a strongly negative impact on patients' quality of life. Therefore, it is important that in our everyday clinical practice, patients who come to our attention suffering from cystitis should not be underestimated. These patients need proper assessment, following specific guidelines since the initial assessment, to prevent misdiagnosis, understand pathophysiology that often is associated with comorbidities, and consequently avoid wrong therapies that can increase risk of recurrence, chronicity, and complications. The purpose of this book is to fill the gaps in the recent literature and provide a guide for daily clinical practice for the clinical assessment of the cystitis and, in relation to therapy, to describe all the available options, including those suggested by the recent research. Some recently introduced therapies are not available in all medical centers; patients' refractory to first-line therapeutic approaches should be referred, when indicated, to hospitals or medical centers that can provide a recommended treatment.

Author details

Giovanni Palleschi
Hemodialysis Unit, Nefrocenter, Frascati, Rome, Italy

*Address all correspondence to: giovanni.palleschi@santagostino.it

References

[1] Bader MS, Loeb M, Leto D, Brooks AA. Treatment of urinary infections in the era of the era of antimicrobial resistance and new antimicrobial agents. Postgraduate Medicine. 2020;**132**(3):234-250. DOI: 10.1080/00325481.2019.1680052 Epub 2019 Oct 24

[2] Colgan R, Williams M. Diagnosis and treatment of acute uncomplicated cystitis. American Family Physician. 2011;**84**(7):771-776

[3] Soytas M, Kactan C, Guven S. Recurrent bladder cystitis: Who takes the role. World Journal of Urology. 2020;**38**(11):2755-2760

[4] Marcu I, Campian EC, Tu FF. Interstitial cystitis/bladder pain syndrome. Seminars in Reproductive Medicine. 2018;**36**(2):123-135. DOI: 10.1055/s-0038-1676089 Epub 2018 Dec 19

[5] Smit SG, Heyns CF. Managment of radiation cystitis. Nature Reviews. Urology. 2010;**7**(4):206-214. DOI: 10.1038/nrurol.2010.23 Epub 2010 Mar 9

Chapter 2

Recurrent Cystitis in Women: Optimal Recommended Diagnostic Evaluation, Management and Prevention Options

Skander Essafi, Maha Abid, Sana Rouis and Amel Omezzine Letaief

Abstract

Cystitis is a very common infection of the lower urinary tract. Women are typically affected, and more than 30 percent will experience at least one episode of cystitis in their lifetime. The diagnosis of this condition and its management are widely known and applied in the outpatient healthcare setting. However, recurrent cystitis, associated with a significant morbidity, is more challenging since their diagnostic evaluation, management and prevention differ significantly between disciplines. Several treatment and prevention options are offered to women with recurrent cystitis. Antibiotic prevention and treatment options should not be first-line, given the importance to limit resistance development and efficacy of alternatives in most situations. The proposed chapter is a narrative review on the current state-of-the-art for the diagnostic evaluation, management and prevention of recurrent cystitis, and aims to discuss other issues and aspects that could be addressed for an optimal management of this condition.

Keywords: urinary tract infection, antimicrobial stewardship, prevention and control, microbial drug resistance, anti-bacterial agents

1. Introduction

Urinary tract infections (UTI) are the most common adult bacterial infection in the world [1, 2]. UTI are twice more likely to occur in women than men over all age groups. A third of women are diagnosed with a UTI before the age of 24 years and half develop at least one episode by 35 years of age. Up to 70% of women will suffer from a UTI during their lifetime, and of those, 30% will have recurrent UTIs. Older women are more likely to get a UTI and suffer from recurrence [3, 4]. Interestingly, the majority of women experiencing recurrence do so despite culture directed antibiotic treatment, having no obvious abnormalities in the urinary tract, so-called uncomplicated UTI.

The differentiation between complicated and uncomplicated UTI has clinical importance for evaluation and type of treatment. In general, uncomplicated UTI is present in immunocompetent patients with no anatomical or functional abnormalities in their urinary tract system and host. Multi-Drug Resistant bacteria was added in the recent interdisciplinary guideline as a factor of complicated UTI [5]. The majority of guidelines reported on otherwise healthy non-pregnant women with uncomplicated rUTI or recurrent cystitis (RC).

RC poses significant clinical challenges, has a major impact on quality of life and represents a substantial social cost. This cost is usually shared between the patient as an out-of-pocket payment, and a co-payment or indemnity with an affiliated health insurance. This also depends on the complexity of the case that would require further investigation, treatment and prophylaxis [6]. According to a recent cost analysis in the United States, doctor visit and diagnosis tools for the RC can cost up to USD 700, the full course of acute antibiotics USD 22 on average for simple RC, or USD 3590 for multi-drug resistant RC. However, prophylaxis can cost on average USD 110 [6].

We present in this review an update on RC features of diagnosis, management and prevention in women who have no obvious causal factor for complications.

2. Definition of recurrent cystitis

Contemporary studies and Guidelines define RC in healthy women as: three episodes of acute symptomatic cystitis in the previous 12 months or two episodes within the 6 months. Proof of a positive urine culture, with strain identification and susceptibility pattern, was also frequently incorporated in the definition. At least 2 culture-proven episodes are suggested. The usually accepted threshold of 10^5 CFU/mL could be lower (10^3 CFU/mL) in RC [7, 8]. Equal or more than 10^2 CFU/mL was also associated with a high Positive Predictive Value, in *E. coli* symptomatic acute cystitis and RC [9]. The differentiation between reinfection (different microorganism, more likely >2 week-interval) and persistent infection (same microorganism and < 2 weeks) is not incorporated in definition of RC. However, it's important for clinician to consider reclassifying patient, treated for uncomplicated cystitis, which recur within 2 weeks, as complicated and require further investigation.

2.1 Etiology/pathogenesis

RCs may be caused by one of two mechanisms: repeated ascending infections or chronic/persistent infection in the bladder.

The source of repeated ascending infections, the same as acute UTI, occurs by the endogenous rectal flora via a perineal–urethral route. Bacteria migrate from the gastrointestinal tract into the bladder. Recent researches demonstrate a complex relationship between intestinal, vaginal and urinary microbiome [10].

The second mechanism, persistent infection in the bladder, explains that 48–80% of UTIs observed were due to a relapse with an *E. coli* strain identical to the primary infecting strain [8]. Moreover, antibiotics applied to the perineal area have been shown to be ineffective in reducing the risk of rUTI. The most plausible hypothesis is the survival of bacteria in bladder through the progression of transient intracellular bacterial communities (IBC) into persistent quiescent intracellular reservoirs. In UroPathogenic *Escherichia coli* (UPEC), of the adhesion molecules, type 1 fimbriae are more associated with IBC formation whereas P fimbriae have a close association with pyelonephritis. As shown in animal models, some species of *E. coli* possess the ability to create a state of quiescent infection in the bladder that may be responsible for multiple recurrences [11, 12].

More specifically, polymorphisms between individuals may include differences in blood groups and cell-mediated immunity [9]. The genetic background of susceptibility to rUTI is not fully understood, but remains an important area of investigation. Further investigation in this area may help lead to early identification of adults predisposed to rUTI and prediction of recurrence rates.

2.2 Risk factors

Understanding the risk factors associated with RC can help physicians to tailor prophylactic strategies to effectively reduce the potential for recurrence. Risk factors for RC can be divided into those related to premenopausal women, and those related to postmenopausal women (**Table 1**). The level of evidence for individual proposed risk factors in both groups varies, and myths about risk and erroneous risk-avoidance behaviors persist among both patients and physicians. However, treatment of asymptomatic bacteriuria in patients with RC has been shown to increase the risk of subsequent symptomatic UTI episodes and is therefore not recommended for these patients [11, 13].

Premenopause: Risk factors in premenopausal women include sexual intercourse, the use of spermicides that may alter vaginal pH and thus affect its flora, changes in bacterial flora, history of UTIs during childhood or family history of UTIs. A greater predisposition for vaginal colonization by uropathogens appears to result from genetic predisposition, potentially due to the increased ability of bacteria to adhere to the epithelium due to an increased expression of *E. coli* receptors on epithelial cells. Lack of postcoital urination, vaginal douches, restrictive underwear, and the hygiene and circumcision status of male partners have been proposed as risk factors, but lack an evidence base.

Postmenopause: A history of UTIs during premenopause increases postmenopausal risk of recurrence. Vulvovaginal atrophy is also a risk factor in this group due to the relationship between reduced estrogen and glycogen production and decreased Lactobacilli colonization. In addition, factors such as urinary incontinence, anterior

	Reduced urine flow	Promoted colonization	Facilitated ascent
All age groups	Inadequate fluid intake	Genetic factors (better adherence bacteria/urothelium)	Urinary incontinence
	Urinary outflow obstruction (calculus, stricture)	Antimicrobial (decreases indigenous flora)	Fecal incontinence
	Atonicbladder		
Sexually-active women	High urine residue	Spermicide (increases binding)	Sexualactivity (increases inoculation)
Post menopause		Estrogendepletion (increases binding)	Vaginal and urethral mucosal atrophy
			Catheterization

Table 1.
Risk factors associated with UTIs and RC [11].

vaginal wall prolapse, increased postvoid residual urine volume, and intermittent or permanent urinary catheterization predispose to complicated UTIs. Women aged >70 years have additional risk factors due to institutionalization with increased rates of catheterization, incontinence, prolapse surgery and decreased functional status.

Nomogram for predicting recurrence risk: A recently published study modeled recurrence risk based on two Italian populations from different centers. Using these data, a nomogram was produced to predict the likelihood of 12-month recurrence based on the most important risk factors identified [14].

3. Diagnosis of recurrent cystitis

3.1 Confirmation of the diagnosis

3.1.1 Clinical confirmation

The diagnosis of RC is based on clinical information and history that allow clinician to confirm and ensure proper reasoning of the diagnosis and management.

First of all, it is necessary to collect all relevant information, together with possibly mentioned in previous records, about the medical history (previous UTI episodes in the last years, antibiotics received for UTI or other infections, any chronic condition, including but not limited to immunosuppressive treatment, renal insufficiency, neurogenic bladder, pregnancy, menopause, current sexual intercourse and previous or existing sexually transmitted infections) [15, 16]. Some factors need to be taken into account, despite not having been largely described in the literature, such as anxiety and emotional disorders, that seem to interfere with complete voiding [17].

Furthermore, anamnesis should be conducted to put the episode of cystitis in its context, including the symptoms that are observed (dysuria, hematuria, nocturia, urgency) as these can predict the positivity of urine cultures, increasing the probability of having a UTI, however there is not a symptom that rules in exclusively the diagnosis of RC [18]. Anamnesis, as well as the physical examination (general, neurological, renal, vaginal), are also important to remove suspicions of other diagnostics, structural abnormality or altered associated comorbidities [16]. Intuitively, it is possible to confirm the diagnosis of recurrent bacterial cystitis based on the definition mentioned above [8].

3.1.2 Urinalysis and urine culture

The prescription of urine dipstick and urine culture varies across guidelines, which may differentiate the entity 'culture proven episodes of acute bacterial cystitis and associated symptoms' [5]. Most recent guidelines except the UK National Institute for Clinical Healthcare and Excellence (NICE) emphasized the importance of urine cultures for the initial diagnosis of RC [19, 20].

In general, both urine examination and urine culture contribute to the diagnosis of RC [5]. In fact, the urine culture often clarifies doubts regarding urine analysis results accuracy. On the other hand, urine analysis can rapidly facilitate the diagnosis and help the clinician, in relatively frequent occurring, with false positive and contaminated urine culture. Combining results of both tests can improve the authenticity of the diagnosis [21]. For the diagnosis of each acute RC episode, guidelines were variable. While it has been shown useful in some recommendations to prescribe dipstick and culture for each acute episode, the EAU and AAFP indicated that repeated urine culture is usually not required if typical symptoms are present and patients are appropriately responding to antibiotics. They should also be performed at least once when the patient is symptomatic [16].

In the case of persistence of symptoms of UTI following a confirmed diagnosis of RC and appropriate use of antimicrobials, some situations are to be considered [22]:

- If the urine culture was positive, and it becomes negative, it may be normal to have ongoing symptoms due to the hypersensitivity of the bladder, especially after a severe UTI episode, and it can be associated with a dysfunction of the pelvic muscle floor. Therefore, the treatment is focused on prevention and hygienic lifestyle (i.e., heading 5. prevention).

- If the urine culture was initially negative or not performed, and/or other symptoms are associated such as microhaematuria $\pm$ micropyuria, other investigations should be performed in order to rule out other diagnostics (i.e., heading 3.a.iii further investigations).

It is widely known that RC culture analyses isolate negative gram rods largely dominated by *E. coli*, followed by *Staphylococcus saprophyticus*, *Proteus mirabilis*, and *Klebsiella pneumoniae* [11].

3.1.3 Further investigations

RC does not require extensive investigations apart from the urine analysis [8]. Cystoscopy and imaging should only be performed without delay in atypical cases, for example, if renal calculi, outflow obstruction, interstitial cystitis or urothelial cancer is suspected [15]. Furthermore, cystoscopy should be recommended also in women that are suspected to suffer from trigonitis. The term "trigonitis" was first introduced in the literature in 1905 as cystitis trigoni [23]. In fact, the reason behind the distinct trigonal endoscopic findings in trigonitis and its underlying pathophysiology is poorly understood. Cystoscpic evaluation is sufficient for the diagnosis and subsequent management of these patients [24]. Endoscopic findings in trigonitis reveal inflammatory lesions such as cystitis cystica, cystitis glandularis, and occasionally small tiny stones within the triangular boundaries of the trigone. Numerous therapeutic strategies have been reported to treat symptomatic trigonitis, including antibiotic therapy, intravesical instillation of different agents, electrofulguration and laser coagulation [25–27].

Further investigation and referral to specialists are indicated in these situations [19].

The SOGC and AWMF guidelines recommend cystoscopy and upper tract imaging in patients with hematuria and persistent urine culture of bacteria other than *E coli* (expert opinion; insufficient evidence) [8].

4. Management of recurrent cystitis

RC leads to a regular consumption of antimicrobials. The choice of antimicrobial therapy is guided by three parameters: efficacity, tolerability, and ecological impact on the gut microbiota [28]. On the other hand, cystitis can be treated with non-antimicrobial treatments of proven efficacy.

4.1 Antimicrobial treatment and stewardship

Without treatment, recurrent cystitis occurring in women with no risk factors of complication is often self-limiting over time and rarely associated with serious complications [29]. However, antimicrobial treatment usually improves symptoms and eliminates bacteria within a few days [30]. Hence, patients with RC should be treated during symptomatic episodes, with an Antimicrobial.

Oral treatment with Fosfomycin-trometamol, Pivmecillinam and nitrofurantoin should be considered for first line treatment, when available. Alternative antimicrobials including trimethoprim alone or combined with a Sulphonamide (Co-trimoxazole) or trimethoprim should only be considered as drugs of first choice in areas with known resistance rates for *E. coli* of <20% [15].

In fact, due to the increasing prevalence of multiresistant bacteria, it is capital to avoid antimicrobial overprescribing. Especially, it is important to save antimicrobials that induce the emergence of antimicrobial resistance, such as the so-called "critically important antimicrobials" [31].

4.1.1 Antimicrobial resistance

Antimicrobial resistance is now one of the most major threats to patient safety worldwide [32]. Resistance to amoxicillin is now 79.8% among urinary isolates of *E. coli* in some countries in Africa, and high levels of resistance to many commonly prescribed antimicrobials have been identified worldwide [33]. More than 20% of *E. coli* strains causing uncomplicated cystitis are now resistant to these agents in several regions of the United States and other countries [34]. The prevalence of resistance to nitrofurantoin among *E. coli* strains is <5%. However, uropathogens non-*E. coli* are often resistant to it. On the other hand, the overuse of fluoroquinolones, antimicrobials that induce the emergence of antimicrobial resistance created resistance to these drugs in UPEC. This resistance is particularly marked in developed countries (55–85% of resistance), compared with developing countries (5–30% of resistance) [35].

Three-day dosing regimens are recommended because of their association with better adherence, lower cost, and lower frequency of adverse reactions, compared to 7–10 day regimens [36]. Several studies confirmed the efficacy of the dosage regimens of 3 days of trimethoprim (TMP), trimethoprim-sulfamethoxazole (TMP-SMX), or a fluoroquinolone for taking management of acute uncomplicated cystitis [36]. By comparison, three-day beta-lactam regimens are less effective than ≥5 days of treatment [36]. Nitrofurantoin is a safe and effective agent but should be administered for a minimum of 7 days. The equivalence of the efficacy of a five-day treatment at nitrofurantoin and a 3-day course of TMP-SMX has been demonstrated [37]. Among other reasonable empirical choices in terms of uncomplicated cystitis, there is also the administration of a single dose of Fosfomycin [36]. The single-dose regimens are less effective than schemas dosages of three to 7 days, even with fluoroquinolones [36, 38]. However, fluoroquinolones can become a reasonable first-line treatment for women in whom the presence of resistance to antimicrobials or an allergy or intolerance to more conventional treatment is confirmed or suspected, as well as for women living in areas where resistance to TMP-SMX is <20% [36].

4.1.2 Side-effects of antimicrobials

Antimicrobial associated collateral damage is critical, producing long-term side effects in the individual patient as well as society as a whole. Several studies have shown that fluoroquinolones and cephalosporins are more likely than other classes of antimicrobials to alter fecal microbiota, and cause *Clostridium difficile* infection and other damage. In fact, fluoroquinolones should not be used to treat acute uncomplicated cystitis because the disabling and serious adverse effects result in an unfavorable risk-benefit ratio [15, 39]. On the other hand, pivmecillinam has an unknown safety profile and potential carnitine deficiency with prolonged use, especially in prophylaxis [40].

4.1.3 Current guidelines for the management of cystitis

The literature search showed that there are several available guidelines affording recommendations for the management of recurrent cystitis. All guidelines recommended short (< 7 days) courses of antimicrobials for treatment of acute episodes in those with recurrent cystitis, rather than prolonged courses [8].

The guidelines of the European Association of Urology (EAU) provided an updated table recapitulating the first-line treatments and alternatives together with the daily dose and the duration of the therapy for recurrent cystitis [15] (**Table 2**). The EAU guidelines strongly recommend not to use aminopenicillins or fluoroquinolones to treat uncomplicated cystitis. However, fluoroquinolone can be prescribed when the use of other antibiotics recommended for the treatment of these infections is considered inappropriate [15].

The **Table 3** showed a comparison of the different guidelines: AUA/CUA/SUFU, SOGC and AAFP [8]. Symptomatic management with analgesia in patients with suspected cystitis is supported by the AUA/CUA/SUFU (while awaiting results of

Antimicrobial	Daily dose	Therapy duration
First line women		
Fosfomycin-trometamol	3 g SD	1
Nitrofurantoin macrocristal	50–100 mg q.i.d.	5
Nitrofurantoin monohydrate/macrocrystal	100 mg b.i.d.	5
Nitrofurantoin microcrystal ER	100 mg b.i.d.	5
Pivmecillinam	200 mg t.i.d	3–5
Alternatives		
Cephalosporins (eg, cefadroxil)	500 mg b.i.d.	3
If the local resistance pattern for E. coli is <20%		
Trimethoprim	200 mg b.i.d	5
Trimethoprim-sulfamethoxazole	160–180 mg b.i.d	3

b.i.d. = bis in die (twice a day); EAU = European Association of Urology; q.i.d. = quarter in die (four times a day); SD = single dose.

Table 2.
First-line treatments and alternatives together with the daily dose and the duration of the therapy for cystitis recommended by the EAU [15].

Issue/ recommendation	EAU*2022	AUA/CUA/SUFU** 2019	SOGC 2010***	AAFP 2016****
Expectant management of recurrent cystitis with analgesia	Antibiotics are recommended but can consider symptomatic therapy in consultation with patient	Likely underutilized, can attempt whilst awaiting cultures	—	Immediate antibiotics leads to better clinical outcomes and delaying antibiotics whilst awaiting cultures is not recommended
Recommend a short course of antibiotic treatments (no longer than 7 days)	Recommend short courses in uncomplicated cystitis nitrofurantoin and fosfomycin-trometamol as first-line antibiotics	Moderate recommendation, evidence level B nitrofurantoin and fosfomycin-trometamol as first-line antibiotics cotrimoxazole among the first-line antibiotics, with the condition " dependent on the local antibiogram "	Recommended antibiotics for a duration of up to 7 days	- Recommend a short course of antibiotics
Recommend self-initiated acute treatment for compliant patients	Strong recommendation	Moderate recommendation	Moderate recommendation	Offer for those who decline prophylactic antibiotics

European Association of Urology. American Urology Association/Canadian Urology Association/ Society of Urodynamics, Female Pelvic Medicine and Urogenital Reconstruction.***Society of Obstetricians and Gynecologists of Canada.****American Academy of Family Physicians.*

Table 3.
Comparison of guidelines' key recommendations on the diagnosis and initial management of recurrent cystitis [8].

urine culture) and SSGO (delay antibiotics for 48 hours and administer analgesia in non-pregnant women aged <65 years with uncomplicated cystitis). Likewise, the NICE guidelines advise on symptomatic management for all patients, but recommended immediate antimicrobials for non-pregnant women, either immediately or deferred if stable or worsening symptoms after 48 h.

Both the AUA/CUA/SUFU and EAU guidelines advocate nitrofurantoin and fosfomycin-trometamol as first-line antimicrobials for the treatment of symptomatic cystitis. The AUA/CUA/SUFU guidelines also include cotrimoxazole among the first-line antimicrobials, with the condition "dependent on the local antibiogram for the treatment of symptomatic cystitis in women", without specifying whether this refers to the patient's antibiogram or the local resistance model [41]. Of the old antimicrobials, the EAU guidelines also include pivmecillinam, an effective molecule according to systematic reviews and meta-analyses [15, 42].

In patients with good compliance, self-diagnosis and self-treatment with a short course regimen of an antimicrobial agent should be considered [15, 42]. The choice of antimicrobials is the same as for sporadic acute uncomplicated cystitis. It is important to notice that patients with recurrent cystitis, developing acute urinary tract infection while receiving antibiotic prophylaxis, should be treated with an alternative Antimicrobial according to the antibiogram.

4.2 Non-antibiotic treatment

We are encountering a real rise in rates of resistance to antimicrobials to undesirable levels worldwide; and untreatable cystitis presents a real concern. This problem is exacerbated by the overuse of antimicrobials. To control this crisis in antimicrobial resistance, nonantimicrobial approaches may be a very interesting alternative to reduce symptoms in acute uncomplicated cystitis without recurring to antimicrobial use [43].

4.2.1 Nonsteroidal anti inflammatorics (NSAIDs)

No studies evaluating NSAIDs as a curative and prophylactic agent for RC have been conducted. However, two randomized controlled trials have evaluated the use of the NSAID (Ibuprofen) for the treatment of acute uncomplicated cystitis in women with interesting results [44, 45].

4.2.2 Chinese herbal medicine (CHM)

The biological plausibility of CHM for recurrent cystitis is supported by in vitro research suggesting that some commonly used Chinese herbs may confer significant diuretic, antibiotic, immune enhancing, antipyretic, anti-inflammatory and, pain-relieving activities for the treatment of recurrent cystitis [46]. Individual herbs such as Huang Lian (Coptis Chinensis Franch) have large spectrum antibacterial activity but also display specific action against *E. coli* [47]. There is growing evidence that some herbal medicines can disable bacterial efflux pumps, and may serve as an important adjuvant treatment to conventional antibiotics [48].

In a recent Meta-analysis comparing the overall effectiveness of treatments during acute phases of infection and rates of recurrence, CHM had a higher rate of effectiveness for acute cystitis (RR 1.21, 95% CI 1.11 to 33) and reduced recurrent cystitis rates (RR 0.28, 95% CI 0.09 to 0.82). Active CHM treatments were more effective in reducing infection incidence (RR 0.40, 95% CI 0.21 to 0.77) [49]. However, the evidence in the premenopausal women is limited. For these reasons, the use of CHM cannot be recommended until larger, and well-conducted randomized trials are performed.

4.2.3 Follow-up

Post-treatment urine cultures in asymptomatic patients are not indicated (**Figure 1**).

RC occurring during the first 2 weeks after treatment of an acute episode suggests a possible relapse and should be managed with pre-treatment urine culture, determination of antimicrobial susceptibility, and treatment with fluoroquinolone for 7 days [15, 28, 38]. Clinical monitoring only is required, and a urine culture should still be performed in case of clinical failure [15, 28].

5. Prevention of recurrent cystitis

Antibiotics are usually effective in the management of acute infections and are the primary means of prophylaxis for patients who experience RC. However, their value is diminished by the emergence of increasing drug-resistant bacteria. Therefore, it is important to develop alternative prevention strategies.

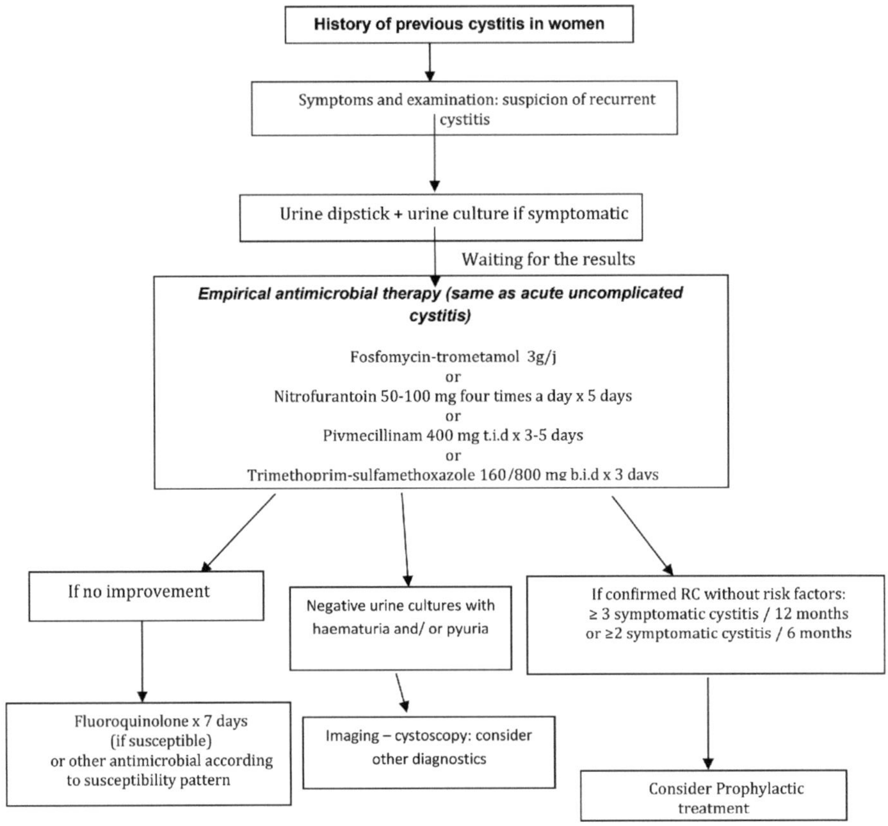

Figure 1.
Algorithm of management of recurrent cystitis.

5.1 Hygienic and dietary measures

Given the stepwise passage of intestinal germs the perineum, then towards the bladder by migrating through the urethra, it is accepted that a simple daily washing of the vulva limits proliferation. Washing before and after sexual intercourse (for both partners) and post-coital micturition can reduce the occurrence of post-coital cystitis [50]. According to the same study, daily changes of underwear also have a significant impact on the accumulation of bacteria in the vulvar region. An interesting British study on post-void wiping habits shows that the directions of the toilet paper have a significant impact on the risk of developing a UTI [51]. It is strongly recommended to wipe from front to back, which is not the case in most countries. This is not the case in almost 50% of this panel of women.

Hydration: The flow of urine mechanically slows down the migration of bacteria to the bladder. It is therefore necessary to diuresis (2 L/day) by sufficient and regular water intake in accordance with the recommendations of the European Food Safety Authority (EFSA) [52], as well as good voiding habits (C-III) [53]. It has been shown that effective flushing of the urinary tract through urine is essential to reduce the uropathic load, provided that bladder emptying is regular and complete provided that regular and complete emptying of the bladder is achieved [54].

Micturition habits: It is essential that micturition is regular. Some micturition habits are unsuitable because they are insufficient (<5 micturitions/d) often because some women hold back. A simple micturition calendar could then be set up over a few days to visualize the micturition calendar the rhythm of micturition and thus to regularize it. In some cases, a voiding reprogramming can be considered. This consists of imposing regular micturition at fixed times initially, then adapted to the diuresis and needs. The regulation of intestinal transit is recommended by professional agreement as a prophylactic measure in the recommendations of the French Agency for Health Products Safety (Afssaps) [55].

Contraception: Women suffering from RC who use a contraceptive method containing a spermicide should be offered an alternative form of contraception.

These conservative measures may be advised, although the evidence is inconclusive.

5.2 Non-antimicrobial prophylaxis

The rationale behind non antimicrobial therapy results from two main drawbacks of the antimicrobial prophylaxis: (i) the emergence of resistant strains in the urine and (ii) the failure to fully eradicate microorganisms with antimicrobial therapy in RC.

5.2.1 Cranberries

Cranberry (in Latin, vaccinium macrocarpon) has attracted a great interest in medical research. The effects of proanthocyanidins (PACs), active constituents inhibiting the adhesion of *E. coli* to uroepithelial cells, have been studied or mentionedin a multitude of publications. It appears that their efficacy, even if controversial, have been shown to be effective in recurrence of cystitis in 20–50% of cases [56]. Cranberry was been shown to be associated to a significant antibiotic consumption decrease. In fact, compliance seems to be better in capsule or powder form (capsules) than in juice. The minimum effective daily dose would be 36 mg of PACs [56, 57]. The duration of action of the active ingredient is proportional to the ingested dose. Thus, 36 mg of PACs twice a day would be preferable for a more prolonged anti-adhesion effect [58]. Cranberry has no significant contraindications. However, there are some undesirable effects, particularly at high doses [57]. The most frequent observed side effects include: episodes of nausea and gastro-esophageal reflux, infrequent, with cranberry juice; mild laxative effects; increased risk of stones with long-term intake in capsule. It should be noted that the consumption of cranberries is contraindicated in the case of treatment with warfarin. A recent Cochrane review of 10 studies with a total of 1049 participants found some evidence that cranberry juice and its derivatives may reduce the number of symptomatic UTIs over a 12-month period, particularly in women who experience RC [59]. Furthermore, there are no definitive data on the amount and the duration of administration for the intervention to reach its maximum effectiveness. Recent data from guidelines showed that experts and panels continue to recommend cranberries for the prophylaxis of RC (Grade C) [60].

5.2.2 D-mannose

Normally present in the human metabolism, D-mannose is involved in the glycolysis of proteins. This simple monosaccharide, naturally found in various plants, and fruits/berries, have the potential to inhibit bacterial adhesion to uroepithelial. Research suggests that free D-mannose in urine saturate *E. coli* FimH structures, and subsequently block *E. coli* adhesion to urinary tract epithelial cells. This so-called competitive inhibition is considered as one of the potential mechanisms for preventing UTI development. In fact, type 1 pili mediate binding, invasion, and biofilm formation of UPEC in the host urothelium during urinary tract infection via the adhesinFimH. Although type 1 fimbriae were extensively studied in *E.coli*, type 1 pili have been documented in several other uropathogens commonly involved in RC, for example, *Klebsiella pneumoniae*. Furthermore, D-mannose does not present an antibiotic-like activity, considering that it does not induce FimH variants that can modify bacterial adhesiveness.

The overall picture of clinical studies with D-mannose in the prophylaxis of RC is favorable. In an open-label clinical trial conducted on 308 women, 3 groups of women over 6 months were compared against the control group, D-mannose (2 g powder/d) provided the same result as daily nitrofuratoin (50 mg/d) [61]. Thus, the risk of recurrence of UTI was reduced by 45%. In addition, the antibiotic caused more adverse events (29%: diarrhea, nausea, skin rush, headache, vaginal burning), whereas D-mannose induced only a few episodes of diarrhea in 8% of cases. However, not many scientific papers advise a daily prophylactic dose of 2 to 3 g of D-mannose. No side effects have been reported [37, 62]. NICE warns takers of cranberry products or D-mannose for the sugar content of these products, which should be considered as part of the person's daily sugar intake [19]. Yet, the quality of studies interested on D-mannose leaves something to be desired; they are mostly confounded with other active ingredients, have small numbers of participants, are open label or uncontrolled.

5.2.3 Vaginal estrogen

Overall, commonly prescribed forms of vaginal estrogen with contemporary dosing schedules can prevent UTIs in postmenopausal women with RC. As a result, the AUA guidelines recommend in peri- and post-menopausal women with RC, clinicians should recommend vaginal estrogen therapy to reduce the risk of future UTIs if there is no contraindication to estrogen therapy (Moderate Recommendation; Evidence Level: Grade B) [8]. However, according to all current guidelines, clinicians should not recommend systemic estrogen to reduce the risk of RC in postmenopausal women.

Data from two small randomized controlled trials indicate that in postmenopausal women with recurrent UTI, the administration of vaginal estrogen results in fewer UTIs [63, 64]. However, there is no sufficient data to recommend one type or form of vaginal estrogen. Creams are less expensive than rings and tables, and may be more effective but they may also be more difficult to apply for some women and may have some side effects (itching, burning, occasional spotting) [62, 63].

5.2.4 Methenamine hippurate

Methenamine Hippurate is a urinary antiseptic agent that is converted to formaldehyde in an acidic urine environment which is directly toxic to bacteria. A randomized control trial in 2022 demonstrated Methenamine Hippurate was non-inferior to prophylactic antibiotics for reducing the incidence of symptomatic UTIs over a 12-month period. Continuous methenamine prophylaxis avoids the risks of long-term prophylactic antibiotic treatment including the development of antibiotic resistance. NHS guidelines recommends that Methenamine might be appropriate for women with a history of RC, given the demonstration of non-inferiority to daily antibiotic prophylaxis seen in various studies [65].

5.2.5 Glycosaminoglycan (GAG) therapy

Exogenous GAGs especially in the combination of HA + CS were investigated for efficacy in preventing RC. Various studies demonstrated intravesical GAGs reduced the recurrence of UTIs caused by *E. coli* and showed clinical benefit up to 36 months after treatment. A randomized double-blind controlled trial of HA + CS + CaCl (four instillations at weekly intervals then five instillations at monthly intervals) monitored for 12 months and patients treated with GAGs therapy had fewer RC and a longer interval free from recurrence [66]. However, the high cost of this treatment still represents a limit, especially with intravesical instillations.

5.2.6 Probiotics

Instillation of Lactobacillus in the vagina is considered to stop the ascent of uropathogens into the bladder. A randomized trial compared high-dose cranberry with Lactobacillus and vitamin A to placebo, and provided low-strength evidence that fewer patients had UTI recurrences with treatment (9.1% versus 33.3%, $p = 0.0053$) [67]. The available studies suggest that probiotics may be beneficial and most authors consider this approach to be promising, but further research is required before probiotics can be recommended for use in the prevention of UTIs.

5.2.7 Immunoprophylaxis: vaccines

Injectable and oral vaccines have been developed in the last decades and shown to be effective and not associated with any observable adverse effects in pregnant women and their offspring [68]. In order to eliminate some of the adverse reactions of the parenteral vaccine, four mucosal vaccines have been developed in the form of a vaginal suppository or oral tablet form; however, the benefits of the vaccine appeared to wane following the last dose [69]. The safety of the only parenteral vaccine currently under development (FimCH) has been proven safe in a Phase I clinical trial. A recent meta-analysis showed that OM-89 (Uro-Vaxom®) showed the greatest reduction in UTI recurrence with a maximum effect shown at 3 months compared with 6 months (RR = 0.67, 95% CI 0.57–0.78). Recent guidelines recommend the use of OM-89 oral vaccine as prophylaxis for RC (Moderate to strong recommendation) [8, 68].

5.2.8 Acupuncture

Two small trials have evaluated the role of acupuncture, compared to placebo acupuncture or no treatment, in the prophylaxis of RC. Over a six-month period, both studies showed that acupuncture could play a significant role in the prevention of RC. They concluded that acupuncture appeared to be a valid alternative to the antibiotic strategy [70].

5.3 Antimicrobial prophylaxis

5.3.1 Prophylactic antibiotics

There are many antimicrobial options for the prevention of RC. A Cochrane review of 19 trials indicated that antibiotics were more effective than placebo in reducing the number of clinical and microbiological recurrences in premenopausal and postmenopausal women with RC [38, 42]. Studies comparing intermittent (post coital) with continuous strategies revealed equal effectiveness. NICE has licensed Nitrofurantoin and Trimethoprim for the prophylaxis of RC. However, all antibiotics have potential risks that should be discussed with patients prior to prescribing for short-, medium-, or long-term prophylaxis. The most tested schedule of antibiotic prophylaxis (TMP, TMP-SMX, nitrofurantoin, cephalexin) was daily dosing. However, Fosfomycin used prophylactically is dosed every 10 days. The duration of antibiotic prophylaxis in the literature ranged from 6 to 12 months. In clinical practice, the duration of prophylaxis can be variable, from 3 to 6 months to 1 year, with periodic assessment and monitoring. Some women stay on continuous or post-coital prophylaxis for years to maintain the benefit without adverse events. However, it should be noted that continuing prophylaxis for years is not evidence-based. The choice of antibiotic should be based on community resistance patterns, adverse events and local costs.

The three main management strategies generally considered are continuous antimicrobial prophylaxis, post-coital prophylaxis and self-treatment patient [38, 42].

5.3.2 Continuous antimicrobial prophylaxis

Continuous prophylaxis can be administered daily at bedtime. Some authors suggest prophylaxis every second night or three nights a week. One study showed that weekly prophylaxis was more effective than monthly prophylaxis. No studies have compared daily and weekly prophylaxis [71]. No recommendation can be made as to the optimal prophylaxis.

5.3.3 Post coital antimicrobial prophylaxis

A causal relationship between infections and sexual intercourse may be suspected when the interval is consistently between 24 and 48 hours [38]. Two studies suggest that in sexually active women experiencing a UTI associated with sexual intercourse the post-coital approach may be a better option [72]. In fact, antibiotic prophylaxis taken before or after sexual intercourse has been shown to be effective and safe. This use of antibiotics is associated with a significant reduction in recurrence rates. Additionally, intermittent dosing is associated with decreased risk of adverse events including gastrointestinal symptoms and vaginitis.

5.3.4 Choice of agents of prophylaxis

For women with RC who are not pregnant, consider a trial of antibiotic prophylaxis only if behavioral and personal hygiene measures, and vaginal estrogen (in postmenopausal women) are not effective or not appropriate [8].

For women with RC; ensure that any current UTI has been adequately treated then consider a trial of daily antibiotic prophylaxis if behavioral and personal hygiene measures alone are not effective or not appropriate, with specialist advice.

Review antibiotic prophylaxis for RC at least every 6 months, with the review to include: assessing the success of prophylaxis; discussion of continuing, stopping or changing prophylaxis (taking into account the person's preferences for antibiotic use and the risk of antimicrobial resistance) (**Table 4**, **Figure 2**).

Antibiotic prophylaxis dosing	
Continuous prophylaxis TMP TMP-SMX Nitrofurantoin Cephalexin Fosfomycin	100 mg once daily 40 mg 200 mg once daily; 40 mg 200 mg thrice weekly 50 mg daily 100 mg daily 125 mg once daily 250 mg once daily 3 g every 10 days
Intermittent prophylaxis TMP-SMX Nitrofurantoin Cephalexin	40 mg 200 mg; 80 mg 400 mg 50 mg; 100 mg 250 mg

Table 4.
Antibiotic prophylaxis dosing for Recurrent Cystitis.

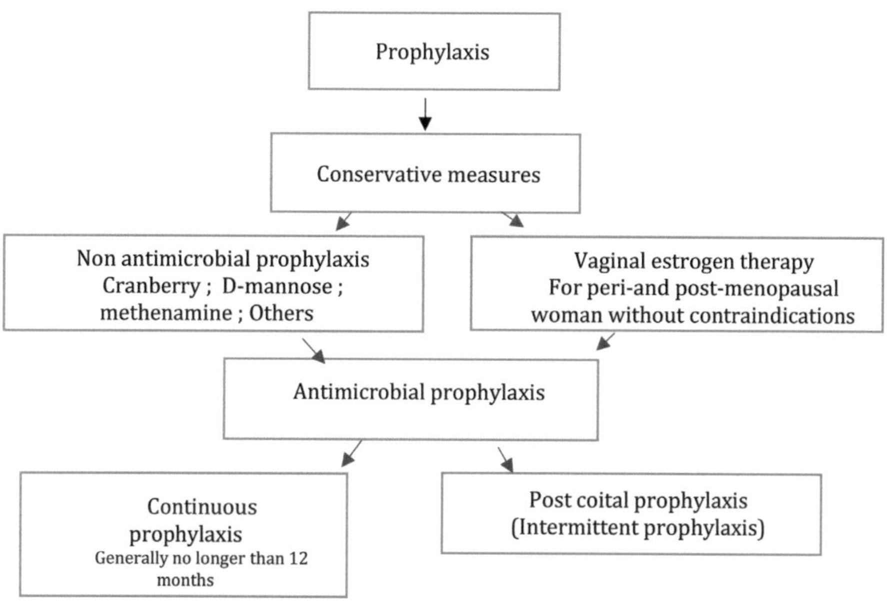

Figure 2.
Prevention algorithm for Recurrent Cystitis.

6. Discussion

This chapter is a narrative review of the current state-of-the-art for the diagnostic evaluation, management and prevention of recurrent bacterial cystitis, and aims to discuss other issues and aspects that could be addressed for the optimal management of this condition.

After a well-conducted anamnesis, the diagnosis of RC should be confirmed. Thus, most recent guidelines emphasized the importance of urine cultures for the initial diagnosis of RC [19, 20]. RC does not require extensive investigations apart from urine analysis and urine culture [8]. Cystoscopy and upper tract imaging are recommended in patients with hematuria and persistent urine culture of bacteria other than E. coli [8]. For the management of RC, antimicrobial treatment usually improves symptoms and eliminates bacteria within a few days. Oral treatment with Fosfomycin-trometamol, Pivmecillinam and nitrofurantoin should be considered for first-line treatment, when available. Alternative antimicrobials including trimethoprim alone or combined with a Sulphonamide (Co-trimoxazole) should only be considered as drugs of first choice in areas with known resistance rates for *E. coli* [15].

Although prophylactic antibiotics remain the preferred preventive treatment in rUTIs, the emergence of antimicrobial resistance worldwide has made the development of non-antibiotic strategies a priority. In this review, we discussed vaccines, D-mannose, Vaginal estrogen, Methenamine Hippurate, Glycosaminoglycan (GAG) therapy, probiotics, bacteriophages, and acupuncture, highlighting the challenges each of these approaches face. Lactobacillus-containing products and cranberry products in conjunction with propolis have shown the most robust results to date and appear to be the most promising new alternative to currently used antibiotics. On another side, proper bladder management is crucial. Women suffering from RC should improve the voiding patterns before or after intercourse and the frequency of urination, ensure good hydration and change contraception based on spermicide. They also should be advised to follow some hygienic measures e.g. avoid the use of hot tubs and tight clothing, although evidence is inconclusive.

7. Future perspectives

A better understanding of UTIs mechanisms will help direct future research on the topic. The nonantibiotic alternatives for rUTI seem promising, but research needs to focus better on the nonantibiotic treatment and prophylaxis of recurrent UTI. Double-blind, placebo-controlled, randomized studies are required to provide high-level evidence of efficacy for all the agents discussed above. A combination of these agents might be the most efficient process to reduce the rate of recurrent UTI without turning to antimicrobial use. Studies of combination therapies in specific patients (such as premenopausal women, postmenopausal women, and men) are also needed to target these treatments optimally. Research into the underlying molecular mechanisms of bacterial adherence and invasion seems most promising and could lead to the identification of novel targets for drug development. These strategies aim to reduce the crisis of antimicrobial resistance and pave the road for a new era in the management of recurrent UTIs.

Abbreviations

AAFP	American Academy of Family Physicians
AUA/CUA/SUFU	Canadian Urological Association (CUA) and Society of Urodynamics, Female Pelvic Medicine and Urogenital Reconstruction (SUFU)
COMEGO	Mexican College of Gynecology and Obstetrics Specialists
EAU	European Society of Urology
NICE	National Institute of Clinical Healthcare and Excellence
RC	Recurrent cystitis
rUTI	Recurrent Urinary Tract Infection
SOGC	Society of Obstetricians and Gynecologists of Canada
SSGO	swiss Society of Gynecology and Obstetrics (SSGO)
SEIMC	Spanish Society of Clinical Microbiology and Infectious Diseases
TMP	trimethoprim
TMP-SMX	trimethoprim-sulfamethoxazole
UPEC	Uropathogenic *E. coli*
UTI	Urinary Tract Infection

Author details

Skander Essafi[1,2*], Maha Abid[3], Sana Rouis[4] and Amel Omezzine Letaief[3]

1 University of Sousse, Tunisia

2 University of Bologna, Italy

3 Farhat Hached Hospital, University of Sousse, Sousse, Tunisia

4 Ibn Jazzar Hospital, University of Sousse, Kairouan, Tunisia

*Address all correspondence to: skander.es@gmail.com

References

[1] Foxman B. Epidemiology of urinary tract infections: Incidence, morbidity, and economic costs. The American Journal of Medicine. 2002;**113** (Suppl 1A):5S-13S

[2] Suskind AM, Saigal CS, Hanley JM, et al. Incidence and Management of Uncomplicated Recurrent Urinary Tract Infections in a National Sample of women in the United States. Urology. 2016;**90**:50-55

[3] Foxman B. Urinary tract infection syndromes: Occurrence, recurrence, bacteriology, risk factors, and disease burden. Infectious Disease Clinics of North America. 2014;**28**:1-13

[4] Glover M, Moreira CG, Sperandio V, et al. Recurrent urinary tract infections in healthy and nonpregnant women. Urological Science. 2014;**25**:1-8

[5] Anger J, Lee U, Ackerman AL, et al. Recurrent uncomplicated urinary tract infections in women: AUA/CUA/SUFU guideline. The Journal of Urology. 2019; **202**:282-289

[6] Gaitonde S, Malik RD, Zimmern PE. Financial burden of recurrent urinary tract infections in women: A time-driven activity-based cost analysis. Urology. 2019;**128**:47-54

[7] Malik RD, Wu YR, Zimmern PE. Definition of recurrent urinary tract infections in women: Which one to adopt? Female Pelvic Medicine & Reconstructive Surgery. 2018;**24**: 424-429

[8] Kwok M, McGeorge S, Mayer-Coverdale J, et al. Guideline of guidelines: Management of recurrent urinary tract infections in women. BJU International. 2022;**130**(Suppl 3):11-22

[9] Hooton TM, Roberts PL, Cox ME, et al. Voided midstream urine culture and acute cystitis in premenopausal women. The New England Journal of Medicine. 2013;**369**:1883-1891

[10] Naboka YL, Mavzyiutov AR, Kogan MI, Gudima IA, Ivanov SN, Naber KG. Does Escherichia coli have pathogenic potential at a low level of bacteriuria in recurrent, uncomplicated urinary tract infection? International Journal of Antimicrobial Agents. 2020; **56**(1):105983. DOI: 10.1016/j.ijantimicag.2020.105983 Epub 2020 Apr 21

[11] Aydin A, Ahmed K, Zaman I, et al. Recurrent urinary tract infections in women. International Urogynecology Journal. 2015;**26**:795-804

[12] Scott VCS, Haake DA, Churchill BM, et al. Intracellular bacterial communities: A potential etiology for chronic lower urinary tract symptoms. Urology. 2015; **86**:425-431

[13] Flores-Mireles AL, Walker JN, Caparon M, et al. Urinary tract infections: Epidemiology, mechanisms of infection and treatment options. Nature Reviews. Microbiology. 2015;**13**: 269-284

[14] Cai T, Mazzoli S, Migno S, et al. Development and validation of a nomogram predicting recurrence risk in women with symptomatic urinary tract infection. International Journal of Urology. 2014;**21**:929-934

[15] EAU Guidelines on Urological Infections - Uroweb. Uroweb - European Association of Urology, Available from: https://uroweb.org/guidelines/urological-infections/summary-of-changes

[16] Dason S, Dason JT, Kapoor A. Guidelines for the diagnosis and management of recurrent urinary tract infection in women. Canadian Urological Association Journal. 2011;**5**:316-322

[17] Ben Hadj Messaoud S, Demonchy E, Mondain V. Recurring cystitis: How can we do our best to help patients help themselves? Antibiot Basel Switz. 2022; **11**:269

[18] Giesen LGM, Cousins G, Dimitrov BD, et al. Predicting acute uncomplicated urinary tract infection in women: A systematic review of the diagnostic accuracy of symptoms and signs. BMC Family Practice. 2010;**11**:78

[19] Overview | Urinary tract infection (recurrent): antimicrobial prescribing | Guidance | NICE, Available from: https://www.nice.org.uk/guidance/ng112 [Accessed: January 7, 2023]

[20] Arnold JJ, Hehn LE et al. Common Questions About Recurrent Urinary Tract Infections in Women. American Family Physician. 2016;**93**(7):560-569

[21] Xie R, Li X, Li G, Fu R. Diagnostic value of different urine tests for urinary tract infection: A systematic review and meta-analysis. Translational Andrology and Urology. 2022;**11**(3):325-335. DOI: 10.21037/tau-22-65

[22] McKertich K, Hanegbi U. Recurrent UTIs and cystitis symptoms in women. Australian Journal of General Practice. 2021;**50**:199-205

[23] Cifuentes L. Epithelium of vaginal type in the female trigone; the clinical problem of trigonitis. The Journal of Urology. 1947;**57**:1028-1037

[24] Engel G, Schaeffer AJ, Grayhack JT, Wendel EF. The role of excretory urography and cystoscopy in the evaluation and management of women with recurrent urinary tract infection. The Journal of Urology. 1980;**123**: 190-191

[25] Hooton TM. Recurrent urinary tract infection in women. International Journal of Antimicrobial Agents. 2001; **17**:259-268

[26] Costantini E, Zucchi A, Del Zingaro M, Mearini L. Treatment of urethral syndrome: A prospective randomized study with Nd: YAG laser. Urologia Internationalis. 2006;**76**: 134-138

[27] Palleschi G, Carbone A, Ripoli A, et al. A prospective study to evaluate the efficacy of Cistiquer in improving lower urinary tract symptoms in females with urethral syndrome. Minerva Urologica e Nefrologica. 2014;**66**:225-232

[28] Caron F, Galperine T, Flateau C, et al. Practice guidelines for the management of adult community-acquired urinary tract infections. Médecine et Maladies Infectieuses. 2018; **48**:327-358

[29] Ferry SA, Holm SE, Stenlund H, et al. The natural course of uncomplicated lower urinary tract infection in women illustrated by a randomized placebo controlled study. Scandinavian Journal of Infectious Diseases. 2004;**36**:296-301

[30] Falagas ME, Kotsantis IK, Vouloumanou EK, et al. Antibiotics versus placebo in the treatment of women with uncomplicated cystitis: A meta-analysis of randomized controlled trials. The Journal of Infection. 2009;**58**: 91-102

[31] World Health Organization. Report of the 1st Meeting of the WHO Advisory

Group on Integrated Surveillance of Antimicrobial Resistance, Copenhagen, 15–19 June 2009. Geneva: World Health Organization; 2011

[32] Akkerman AE, Kuyvenhoven MM, Verheij TJM, et al. Antibiotics in Dutch general practice: Nationwide electronic GP database and national reimbursement rates. Pharmacoepidemiology and Drug Safety. 2008;**17**:378-383

[33] Bryce A, Hay AD, Lane IF, et al. Global prevalence of antibiotic resistance in paediatric urinary tract infections caused by Escherichia coli and association with routine use of antibiotics in primary care: Systematic review and meta-analysis. BMJ. 2016; **352**:i939

[34] Gupta K, Scholes D, Stamm WE. Increasing prevalence of antimicrobial resistance among uropathogens causing acute uncomplicated cystitis in women. JAMA. 1999;**281**:736-738

[35] Kot B. Antibiotic resistance among Uropathogenic Escherichia coli. Polish Journal of Microbiology. 2019;**68**: 403-415

[36] Warren JW, Abrutyn E, Hebel JR, et al. Guidelines for antimicrobial treatment of uncomplicated acute bacterial cystitis and acute pyelonephritis in women. Infectious Diseases Society of America (IDSA). Clinical Infectious Diseases. 1999;**29**: 745-758

[37] Gupta K, Hooton TM, Roberts PL, et al. Short-course nitrofurantoin for the treatment of acute uncomplicated cystitis in women. Archives of Internal Medicine. 2007;**167**:2207-2212

[38] Hooton TM, Stamm WE. Diagnosis and treatment of uncomplicated urinary tract infection. Infectious Disease Clinics of North America. 1997;**11**:551-581

[39] Smith AL, Brown J, Wyman JF, et al. Treatment and prevention of recurrent lower urinary tract infections in women: A rapid review with practice recommendations. The Journal of Urology. 2018;**200**:1174-1191

[40] Morley GL, Wacogne ID. UK recommendations for combating antimicrobial resistance: A review of 'antimicrobial stewardship: Systems and processes for effective antimicrobial medicine use' (NICE guideline NG15, 2015) and related guidance. Archives of Disease in Childhood. Education and Practice Edition. 2017;**103**:46-49

[41] Naber KG, Bonkat G, Wagenlehner FME. The EAU and AUA/CUA/SUFU guidelines on recurrent urinary tract infections: What is the difference? European Urology. 2020;**78**: 645-646

[42] Schaeffer A, J, Stuppy BA. Efficacy and safety of self-start therapy in women with recurrent urinary tract infections. The Journal of Urology. 1999;**161**(1): 207-211

[43] Sihra N, Goodman A, Zakri R, et al. Nonantibiotic prevention and management of recurrent urinary tract infection. Nature Reviews. Urology. 2018;**15**:750-776

[44] Gágyor I, Bleidorn J, Kochen MM, Schmiemann G, Wegscheider K, Hummers-Pradier E. Ibuprofen versus fosfomycin for uncomplicated urinary tract infection in women: Randomised controlled trial. The BMJ. 2015;**351**: h6544

[45] Roy KR, Reddy GV, Maitreyi L, et al. Celecoxib inhibits MDR1 expression

through COX-2-dependent mechanism in human hepatocellular carcinoma (HepG2) cell line. Cancer Chemotherapy and Pharmacology. 2010;**65**:903-911

[46] Huang KC. The Pharmacology of Chinese Herbs. UK: CRC-Press; 1992

[47] Yan D, Jin C, Xiao X-H, et al. Antimicrobial properties of berberines alkaloids in Coptis chinensis Franch by microcalorimetry. Journal of Biochemical and Biophysical Methods. 2008;**70**:845-849

[48] Stavri M, Piddock LJV, Gibbons S. Bacterial efflux pump inhibitors from natural sources. The Journal of Antimicrobial Chemotherapy. 2007;**59**: 1247-1260

[49] Flower A, Wang L-Q, Lewith G, et al. Chinese herbal medicine for treating recurrent urinary tract infections in women. Cochrane Database of Systematic Reviews. 2015;**2015**: CD010446

[50] Badran YA, El-Kashef TA, Abdelaziz AS, et al. Impact of genital hygiene and sexual activity on urinary tract infection during pregnancy. Urology Annals. 2015;7:478-481

[51] Persad S, Watermeyer S, Griffiths A, et al. Association between urinary tract infection and postmicturition wiping habit. Acta Obstetricia et Gynecologica Scandinavica. 2006;**85**:1395-1396

[52] European Food Safety Authority. Scientific opinion on dietary reference values for water. EFSA Journal. 2010; **8**(3):1459

[53] Bruyère F, Cariou G, et al. Cystites aiguës. Progrès en Urologie. 2008;**18** (S1):9-13

[54] Mulvey MA, Schilling JD, Martinez JJ, et al. Bad bugs and beleaguered bladders: Interplay between uropathogenic Escherichia coli and innate host defenses. Proceedings of the National Academy of Sciences of the United States of America. 2000;**97**: 8829-8835

[55] Association française de sécurité sanitaire des produits de santé (Afssaps). Recommandations de bonnes pratiques: diagnostic et antibiothérapie des infections urinaires bactériennes communautaires chez l'adulte. SPILF. 2015

[56] Canadian Task Force on Preventive Health Care. New grades for recommendations from the Canadian task force on preventive health care. Canadian Medical Association Journal. 2003;**169**:207-208

[57] American College of Obstetricians and Gynecologists. ACOG practice bulletin No. 91: Treatment of urinary tract infections in nonpregnant women. Obstetrics and Gynecology. 2008;**111**(3): 785-794

[58] Minardi D, Parri G, d'Anzeo G, et al. Perineal ultrasound evaluation of dysfunctional voiding in women with recurrent urinary tract infections. The Journal of Urology. 2008;**179**:947-951

[59] Jepson RG, Williams G, Craig JC. Cranberries for preventing urinary tract infections. Cochrane Database of Systematic Reviews. 2012;**10**:CD001321

[60] Taich L, Zhao H, Cordero C, Anger JT. New paradigms in the management of recurrent urinary tract infections. Current Opinion in Urology. 2020;**30**(6):833-837

[61] Wright SW, Wrenn KD, Haynes ML. Trimethoprim-sulfamethoxazole resistance among urinary coliform

isolates. Journal of General Internal Medicine. 1999;**14**(10):606-609

[62] Franco AVM. Recurrent urinary tract infections. Best Practice & Research. Clinical Obstetrics & Gynaecology. 2005;**19**:861-873

[63] Perrotta C, Aznar M, Mejia R, et al. Oestrogens for preventing recurrent urinary tract infection in postmenopausal women. Cochrane Database of Systematic Reviews. 2008; **2008**:CD005131

[64] Cardozo L, Lose G, McClish D, et al. A systematic review of estrogens for recurrent urinary tract infections: Third report of the hormones and urogenital therapy (HUT) committee. International Urogynecology Journal and Pelvic Floor Dysfunction. 2001;**12**:15-20

[65] Harding C, Mossop H, Homer T, et al. Alternative to prophylactic antibiotics for the treatment of recurrent urinary tract infections in women: Multicentre, open label, randomised, non-inferiority trial. BMJ. 2022;**376**: e068229

[66] De Vita D, Giordano S. Effectiveness of intravesical hyaluronic acid/ chondroitin sulfate in recurrent bacterial cystitis: A randomized study. International Urogynecology Journal. 2012;**23**:1707-1713

[67] Koradia P, Kapadia S, Trivedi Y, et al. Probiotic and cranberry supplementation for preventing recurrent uncomplicated urinary tract infections in premenopausal women: A controlled pilot study. Expert Review of Anti-Infective Therapy. 2019;**17**: 733-740

[68] Aziminia N, Hadjipavlou M, Philippou Y, et al. Vaccines for the prevention of recurrent urinary tract infections: A systematic review. BJU International. 2019;**123**:753-768

[69] Hopkins WJ, Uehling DT. Vaccine development for the prevention of urinary tract infections. Current Infectious Disease Reports. 2002;**4**: 509-513

[70] Alraek T, Soedal LIF, Fagerheim SU, et al. Acupuncture treatment in the prevention of uncomplicated recurrent lower urinary tract infections in adult women. American Journal of Public Health. 2002;**92**:1609-1611

[71] Ramírez Sevilla C, Gómez Lanza E, Llopis Manzanera J, et al. A focus on long-term follow-up of Immunoprophylaxis to recurrent urinary tract infections: 10 years of experience with MV140 vaccine in a cohort of 1003 patients support high efficacy and safety. Archivos Españoles de Urología. 2022;**75**: 753-757

[72] Stapleton A, Latham RH, Johnson C, et al. Postcoital antimicrobial prophylaxis for recurrent urinary tract infection. A randomized, double-blind, placebo-controlled trial. JAMA. 1990; **264**:703-706

Chapter 3

Cystitis in Children

Dragana Živković and Maja Samardžić Lukić

Abstract

Urinary tract infections in children are very common. However, their etiology, treatment, and prognosis are very different compared to adult patients. It is a field of interest that is covered by Pediatricians, Pediatric Nephrologists, Pediatric Surgeons, and Pediatric Urologists. There are of course different approaches with a common goal of urinary tract treatment, prevention, and in more serious cases kidney function preservation. This chapter offers a comprehensive review on the topic, with an attempt to offer impartial analysis of the practices widely accepted in treatment of urinary tract infections in childhood, with all the specific procedures typical for pediatric population.

Keywords: cystitis, children, vesicoureteral reflux, pyelonephritis, bladder and bowel elimination syndrome

1. Introduction

Cystitis represents a condition in which there is an inflammation of the bladder mucosa, caused by different factors [1]. Modern medical literature is mostly based on cystitis of an infectious etiology, due to its significant frequency in both general and pediatric populations [2, 3]. Nevertheless, it would be wrong to disregard the fact that some forms of cystitis in children could be of non-infectious etiology. They can be acute or chronic, and their clinical manifestations can vary from asymptomatic forms to life-threatening ones [4]. Due to its frequency and a tendency for recurrence, cystitis represents a significant health problem in childhood [1, 2].

Following a large number of publications about cystitis in adults, there has been increasing interest in cystitis in the pediatric population taking into account various causes, as well as the possibility of negative long-term renal consequences and quality of patients' life.

We searched for the available literature to identify studies and reviews relevant to the scope of this review. Considering different epidemiologic aspects of urinary bladder infections, this chapter also represents a summary of international guidelines from pediatric and pediatric urologic societies.

2. Classification and pathogenesis

There are several necessary factors for the development of infectious cystitis: breakthrough of the pathogenic microorganisms into the bladder, as well as their growth and reproduction. As a part of a lower urinary tract infection (LUTI), the bladder is inflamed together with the urethra, but sometimes the entire urinary system is affected irrespective of the point of origin of the infection [2].

The newest classifications of cystitis take into account the clinical presentation and risk factors and are accordingly classified into symptomatic and asymptomatic, i.e. complicated and uncomplicated cystitis [1]. **Symptomatic cystitis** represents a condition with clearly present symptoms related to the lower urinary tract. **Asymptomatic bacteriuria** represents the finding of significant bacteriuria in a child without lower urinary tract symptoms (LUTS). There are a significant number of non-virulent strains of bacteria that do not cause a response activation of the organism. In children with neurogenic bladder, it is sometimes difficult to differentiate between the symptomatic and asymptomatic forms of cystitis [1, 5].

Uncomplicated cystitis develops in children with normal morphologic and functional characteristics of the urinary system, while **complicated cystitis** is defined as an inflammation of the bladder mucosa in children with already present disorders of the urinary system, or associated diseases [5].

3. Epidemiology

The exact incidence of cystitis in children is not determined, as most of the published data in modern literature refer to overall UTI in the pediatric population [3]. Incidence depends on the gender as well as the age of the child. UTI are more common in males only in the newborn period, most likely due to the greater incidence of congenital urinary tract malformations in boys. In children up to two years of age, there is a strong tendency for the infection to spread over the entire urinary system in a very short period. Cystitis then develops as a part of the infection of the entire urinary system, with non-specific clinical presentation. Therefore, cystitis in children often goes unrecognized [3, 5, 6]. From the second year onwards, the incidence of cystitis and UTI, in general, are more common in girls [2]. School-aged girls have a UTI incidence of 1–3%, and with the start of sexual activity, it rises up to 10% [3, 7, 8]. Asymptomatic bacteriuria is more common in school-aged girls [3%] and male newborns (1%) [5].

In the first 6–12 months after the first UTI, approximately 30% of children have a recurrent UTI of different localization. If a recurrence appears, there are several risk factors that need to be evaluated with additional diagnostic procedures [2, 5].

4. Etiology

Different microorganisms can cause cystitis. They are usually an integral part of the normal bowel flora. Less commonly, microorganisms invade the urinary tract system from the environment during different diagnostic and therapeutic procedures [9, 10].

The most common microorganisms causing cystitis in children are **gram-negative** bacteria from the family of Enterobacteriaceae. *Escherichia coli* is the normal inhabitant of the bowel flora and it is a cause of up to 80–90% of all cystitis [2, 10]. It is most commonly diagnosed in uncomplicated cystitis, i.e. in children without congenital malformations, stones, or inserted urinary catheters [3].

Other gram-negative bacteria (Proteus, Klebsiella, Enterobacter, and Pseudomonas) are less common causative agents of cystitis, and they play a role in recurrent infections and infections related to anatomic and functional malformations of the bladder. They are also more commonly associated with urolithiasis and nosocomial infections related to different urological interventions. It is well known that *Proteus mirabilis* and *Klebsiella* are producing urease, extracellular mucus, and polysaccharides that take part in the development of the urinary calculi, and are therefore significant causative agents associated with urolithiasis [2, 3, 10].

Gram-positive bacteria are less relevant in pediatric bladder infections. The most commonly isolated bacteria are coagulase-negative *Staphylococcus saprophyticus*. It is a cause of 10–15% of acute cystitis in adolescent girls [10]. Enterococcus and *Staphylococcus aureus* are isolated in cystitis in patients with urolithiasis, previous urological interventions, or placed urinary catheters. *Ureaplasma urealyticum* is sometimes diagnosed in girls in puberty [2, 10].

Besides bacteria, cystitis might be caused by other microorganisms, but far less commonly. In immunocompromised children, children with diabetes, and children with indwelling catheters colonization of the bladder with Candida and/or other **fungi** is not uncommon. In these cases, one must take into account the risk of the progression of cystitis into an invasive systemic infection, necessitating adequate diagnosis and treatment [2, 11, 12].

Viral cystitis is most commonly diagnosed in patients with bone marrow transplantation. The most common causative agents are viruses from the polyoma group (BK virus, JC virus, and cytomegalovirus) [13]. **Adenovirus** can cause epidemic hemorrhagic cystitis in the pediatric population without comorbidities [10].

Infectious agents	
Bacterial	*Gram-negative:* • *Escherichia coli* • *Proteus* • *Klebsiella* • *Enterobacter* • *Pseudomonas* *Gram-positive:* • *Staphylococcus saprophyticus* • *Staphylococcus aureus* • *Enterococcus* • *Ureaplasma urealyticum* *Mycobacterium tuberculosis*
Viral	Adenovirus BK virus JC virus Cytomegalovirus
Fungi	*Candida*
Parasitical	*Schistosomiasis haematobium*
Non-infectious agents	
Chemical	Medications (e.g. cyclophosphamide)
Allergic	Soap, baths

Table 1.
Etiopathogenic agents of cystitis in children.

Infection of the bladder with **mycobacteria tuberculosis** is a rare, but very serious infection. Unrecognized and inadequately treated, it can have severe complications, such as urinary stricture and decreased bladder compliance [11].

Parasitic causes of cystitis should be suspected in children coming from endemic regions, or bad hygienic conditions. The most commonly diagnosed parasite as a cause of cystitis is *Schistosomiasis haematobium* [10].

There is only a little literature data on **non-infectious cystitis** in children. Certain medications used in pediatric oncology and pediatric immunology are known to cause chemical cystitis [4]. It is proven that cyclophosphamide use can cause Hemorrhagic Cystitis (HC). Adequate hydration as a preventive measure for the development of HC is an important part of supportive therapy in patients treated with cyclophosphamide [14] (read the chapter: ***"Drugs related cystitis"*** of this book).

The use of different soaps and baths in children can cause chemical/allergic reactions when in contact with the urethral mucosa. This reaction can spread upstream to the bladder causing inflammation of the bladder mucosa. This is more common in girls, due to a shorter urethra and consequent faster spread of inflammation [15].

In cases of cystitis caused by a non-infectious agent, urine culture is typically negative. However, sometimes the chemical agent leading to the inflammation of the bladder mucosa serves as a starting point for the colonization of the bladder with bacteria. This is an important fact to be taken into account when diagnosing and treating cystitis (**Table 1**).

5. Pathophysiology

The bladder is the distal part of the urinary system and is a temporary reservoir for collecting urine. The proximal part of the urethra and the bladder are generally sterile. The dominant way of a breakthrough of the microorganisms in this region is the ascending one. In children predisposed to the development of cystitis, the first region that gets colonized is the periurethral region, the vaginal introitus, and the prepuce. Due to the invasion of the microorganisms in this region, subsequently, the bladder mucosa gets inflamed. If, in certain cases, the bladder is infected after the primary infection of the kidneys and upper urinary tract, we refer to that kind of infection as descendent [2, 9, 16].

Many factors enable the development of cystitis, and they represent a good example of interaction between the host and the microorganism. For the development of the infection of the bladder mucosa, the virulence of the microorganism is as important as the sensitivity of the host and its defense mechanisms [16].

The most studied is the virulence of *Escherichia coli* as the most common cause of cystitis. The most important factor determining the virulence of *E. coli* is the existence of the so-called fimbriae—filamentous organelles (P-fimbriae). They enable the bacteria to get attached to the uroepithelium and prevent its flushing with the stream of urine. At the same time, they enable its ascent towards the upper parts of the urinary system. Thanks to the recognition of the fimbria structure, as well as the structure and mechanism of action of the receptors on the urothelium for P-fimbriae and their mechanism of interaction, it is possible to determine in the laboratory setting the existence of this particularly virulent and pathogenic strain of *E. coli*. There are other factors influencing the virulence of *E. coli* such as endotoxin, chymolysine, cytotoxic necrosis factor, as well as the use of different metals (iron and zinc) for nutrition through a system of siderophores and chemoreceptors, the mobility due to flagella existence, and avoidance of the immune response of the host [2, 3, 16].

An important role in the development of cystitis is the disturbance of the general as well as local defense mechanisms of the child. Of the local ones, the most important role is that of the normal urinary hydrodynamic. If due to anatomical or functional disorders there are disturbances in the normal process of urine elimination, the residual urine decreases the normal bactericidal capacity of the uroepithelial cells leading to the fast reproduction of the bacteria [9].

The most common predisposing factors for the development of cystitis are malformations of the urinary tract, primary, and secondary vesicoureteral reflux (VUR), obstructions at different levels and different etiologies, urolithiasis, and different forms of bowel and bladder elimination syndrome [17].

Factors predisposing to the periurethral colonization and disturbance of normal periurethral flora in children, such as previous use of antibiotics for any indication [3], play a special role in the development of cystitis in children. In adolescent girls, the initiation of sexual intercourse plays an important role in the development of cystitis. The use of contraceptives causes changes in the previous vaginal microbial flora, increasing the risk of cystitis development [18].

The presence of a non-retractable prepuce in male infants is a well-documented risk factor for the development of cystitis. It has been shown that uncircumcised infants have a 10 times bigger risk of cystitis development compared to their circumcised counterparts [19].

Congenital or acquired IGA immunodeficiency also contributes to the vulnerability of the pediatric population and their predisposition towards cystitis development. Another group of pediatric populations with an increased incidence of cystitis are patients with diabetes mellitus [2, 3].

There is more and more data corroborating genetic predisposition to cystitis. An important factor in the development of urinary tract infections is the presence of specific receptors on the urothelial cells that are binding with the bacteria. The number and type of those receptors are genetically determined. Most of these structures are parts of blood group antigens that are present on erythrocytes and uroepithelial cells [20]. Genes that might be responsible for the preponderance of recurrent urinary tract infections are HSPA1B, CXCR1, CXCR2, TLR2, TLR4, and TGFbeta1 [21]. Although few significant mutations are identified to implement these data into daily clinical practice, further research is necessary [3].

6. Clinical presentation

Symptoms of cystitis in the pediatric population are different at different ages. In the first months of life, the symptoms of UTI are non-specific, and if not recognized early, they might develop into pyelonephritis and sepsis. Infants with urinary tract infections often present with lethargy, irritability, failure to thrive, and prolonged neonatal jaundice. Sometimes there are also vomiting and diarrhea. Neonate or an infant is usually febrile pointing toward an infection of the upper urinary tract and systemic infection. That is why a UTI should be suspected in every neonate or infant with an unclear cause of fever.

From the age of approximately 3–24 months, the symptoms are similar. Urine might be turbid and malodorous, and a child might be complaining of abdominal pain. After the second year, the symptoms become more specific, similar to symptoms in the adult population. Cystitis is usually manifested with dysuria, urgency, and frequency. Enuresis appears in some cases in children that have previously achieved nocturnal continence. These symptoms are often accompanied by fever up to 38°C, malodorous urine, and macroscopic hematuria [2, 11, 16].

Symptoms and signs of fungal cystitis are very similar. Besides the aforementioned symptoms, anuria might develop as a consequence of the obstruction of the urinary system due to the presence of the so-called "fungal ball" formed in the bladder.

The clinical presentation of viral cystitis essentially does not differ from the presentation of bacterial cystitis. Dysuria, macroscopic hematuria, and suprapubic pain are the most common manifestations of viral cystitis [2, 13].

Differential diagnosis in children when cystitis is suspected could be nephrolithiasis, urinary tract obstruction of different etiologies, appendicitis, gastroenteritis, parasitic bowel infections, vulvovaginitis, and balanitis. In adolescent girls that are sexually active and have cystitis with or without vaginitis, pregnancy should always be considered [22].

7. Diagnosis

Diagnosis of cystitis is based on well-taken patient history, physical examination, and laboratory testing. The patient history should include the question of first or recurrent infections, fetal abnormalities, and any malformations of the urinary tract, prior surgeries, family history, and the presence of obstipation or voiding dysfunctions. The radiologic examination is unnecessary for diagnosing cystitis but is important in the diagnostics of anatomical and functional abnormalities of the urinary tract predisposing to the development of cystitis in children.

Adequate choice of diagnostics is very important for differentiating between infections of the upper urinary tract system (pyelonephritis) and lower urinary tract infection (cystitis), which is often very challenging [23].

The physical examination should include a whole-body examination of the throat, lymph nodes, abdomen, genitalia, flank, and back. It most often reveals abdominal or suprapubic tenderness on palpation. Voiding is interrupted, the flow is weak, and there is straining and decreased voided volume, sometimes up to only a few drops of urine. Examination of the external genitalia might reveal certain anomalies, like the presence of a foreign body, vulvitis, or balanitis, or indicate a possible sexual assault [10, 16].

In acute cystitis, fever might be present, but most of the patients are subfebrile. Systemic laboratory inflammation parameters alone are not sufficient to confirm the presence of cystitis. In circumstances of the negative findings of C reactive protein, procalcitonin pyelonephritis could be excluded [24, 25].

The golden standard in diagnosing UTI, that is, cystitis is significant bacteriuria. To take this finding truly as a golden standard, sampling must be done appropriately. The choice of sampling method depends on the age of the patient, the urgency of the testing, and the need for the microbiological examination. This is particular challenge in non-toilet-trained children. Urine can be obtained with urine sampling bags in neonates and infants, by catching the middle stream of urine during voiding in older children, or in special circumstances by catheterization either suprapubically or through the urethra. Before urine sampling, adequate hygiene of the periurethral region is recommended [11, 22, 26].

A sampling of urine with urine sampling bags is used in children that have not achieved voluntary voiding. The testing of the urine collected in such a way can be only used as a screening method, and further microbiological tests of such urine are not recommended. The American Academy of Pediatrics (AAP) guideline states that bag cultures have "an unacceptably high false-positive rate and are valid only when they yield negative results," stating that the rate of false positives ranges from 88 to 99% of tests [3, 27].

If the chemical and cytological finding of the urine is normal, UTI can be ruled out. In case of a pathological finding, it is necessary to obtain another urine sample some other way due to a high chance of contamination [28].

First-morning urine sampling should be performed in children with voluntary voiding. In toddlers that are still not fully toilet trained, a clean catch might be attempted, in which case a risk of contamination is far less than in urine collected in a sampling urine bag. In any case for the results to be evaluated adequately, the sampling method must be noted [28, 29]. Suprapubic and lumbosacral stimulation are the methods of voiding stimulation. Another alternative is the Quick-Wee method of urine collection. In this method, the suprapubic area stimulated by using a gauze soaked in cold fluid and the voided midstream urine is caught in sterile cup [3, 28].

When it is not possible to collect urine non-invasively then catheter sampling or suprapubic aspiration should be used. Catheterization of the bladder is usually performed in children younger than 3 years. It is considered a safe and reliable urine sampling method, with a low risk of introducing bacteria into the urinary system. Suprapubic aspiration is the most reliable urine sampling method in neonates and infants but is also the most invasive one. It is performed in critically ill children in a need of prompt and reliable diagnostics [28].

After adequate urine sampling, the analysis could be performed with the dipstick test and/or microscopic examination of the urine sediment, and additional microbiological analysis could be performed when needed. The main advantage of the dipstick test is the availability of prompt information that could influence further diagnostics and treatment. The most commonly used findings in a dipstick test are leukocytic esterase and nitrites. Leukocytic esterase is an enzyme produced by leucocytes that can be found in urine during an active bladder infection. Positive leucocyte esterase on a dipstick test corresponds to the finding of more than 5 leukocytes in a microscopic exam. Nitrites are a side product of bacterial metabolism in the bladder. Compared to leukocytic esterase, nitrites are less sensitive, but more specific in diagnosing cystitis. Urine that is left at room temperature for more than 1 hour is not useful, leukocyte esterase test loses sensitivity, and nitrite test loses specificity. Macroscopic or microscopic hematuria is often associated with cystitis, irrespective of positive leukocytic esterase and nitrites [1, 10, 11, 22, 30]. Sterile pyuria may occur in association with infections such as tuberculosis, fungal, viral, and parasitic. It can also occur with acute glomerulonephritis, analgesic nephropathy, appendicitis, or chemical cystitis [3, 10].

Significant bacteriuria is defined as more than 100,000 colony-forming units (CFUs)/mL if urine is collected through the clean catch of the first-morning urine. Since 2011, there has been a recommendation from the AAP that significant bacteriuria in children 2–24 months old is the finding of 50,000 colony-forming units (CFUs)/mL of urine [27]. Finding less than 10,000 colony-forming units (CFUs)/mL of urine is considered contamination. If the urine is obtained through suprapubic aspiration, the finding of any bacteria in urine is significant, and in cases of urine sampling through catheterization, the significant bacteriuria is defined as more than 10,000 colony-forming units (CFUs)/mL of urine. Multiple isolated bacteria suggest contamination of a urine sample. Also, the presence of more than 10 epithelial cells with an insignificant number of bacteria in urine culture suggests contamination.

Non-uropathogenic bacteria are Lactobacillus, *Staphylococcus epidermidis*, and *Streptococcus viridans*. The growth of these bacteria in urine culture is also considered contamination. Patients with urinary frequency (i.e., decreased bladder incubation time) are those most likely to have bacteria proliferating in the urinary bladder in the presence of low colony counts, which can result in false-negative results [3, 11, 23, 31].

To confirm the diagnosis of **candida cystitis,** the finding of more than 10,000/ml of urine is necessary. Since most fungal urinary infections are associated with urinary tract malformations, ultrasound is a very useful diagnostic tool. It is especially useful in identifying "fungus balls" in the bladder [2, 12].

Diagnosis of **viral cystitis** is based upon the identification of the presence of the virus in the urine with PCR. Serologic examinations are unreliable in diagnosing viral cystitis, especially in immunocompromised children, due to an inadequate immune response in such patients [2].

An effort should be made to localize an infection and identify causative organism because some patients do not need conventional antibiotic therapy (viral and chemical cystitis, etc.) [27].

Ultrasound is not a mandatory part of the diagnostic protocol in patients with cystitis. If performed, an ultrasound usually shows thickened bladder wall. In patients with repeated cystitis, it should be done after the acute phase of infection, to avoid false-positive findings associated with edema of the bladder mucosa or dilatation of the urinary tract due to the release of endotoxins. It is, however, mandatory in cases of the suspected presence of urinary tract anomalies, the presence of obstruction, or in cases of recurrent cystitis of unclear etiology [3, 9].

Whatever, in order to make the correct diagnosis of cystitis and make a good decision, it is very important to take into account all the mentioned diagnostic criteria. Taking these parameters in combination can improve the sensitivity and specificity compared with testing each in isolation.

8. Treatment

The treatment of cystitis aims to remove the causative agent of the bladder inflammation and prevent further breakthroughs of the infection, and its recurrence.

Children with cystitis are usually treated ambulatory. In cases of dehydration, intolerance of oral intake, or urinary tract obstruction, it is necessary to admit the patient. Absolute indication for admittance is a neonate and an infant less than 2 months of age with UTI since in those patients there is a high risk of the development of a systemic infection [23, 26, 27].

If a bacterial urinary infection is suspected, empirical antibiotic treatment should be started as soon as possible. In most cases, before the start of the therapy, the exact causative agent and its sensitivity to antibiotics are not known. Treatment should start after sampling the urine for urine culture. The choice of antibiotic should be based on the knowledge of the local epidemiological situation, primarily regarding any resistance to antibiotics. In the treatment of isolated cystitis, oral antibiotics are prescribed to all patients that can tolerate oral intake [1, 3, 32]. Parenteral antibiotics are prescribed to patients with vomiting and dehydration. Most of the treatment guides for the treatment of UTI in children recommend cephalosporins of the first and second generation, amoxicillin-clavulanic acid, and nitrofurantoin [3, 11, 22, 23]. Due to the high incidence of resistance, certain guidelines do not recommend the use of trimethoprim-sulfamethoxazole as an empiric therapy except in cases when the sensitivity to this antibiotic is confirmed with an antibiogram. If urine culture shows that an empirically chosen antibiotic is not appropriate for that infection, in case of a clinical improvement the chosen antibiotic should be continued [26, 33].

The use of ciprofloxacin in the pediatric population is controversial and justified only when there is a severe clinical form of the infection, and there is no other antibiotic to which a particular bacterial strain is sensitive. It should be taken into account the fact that due to the frequent use of those antibiotics in the adult population, there is increased resistance to this group of antibiotics [34, 35].

Short-term antibiotic treatments are becoming more popular, due to better compliance, decreased expenses, and decreased incidence of antibiotic side effects. Most of the guidelines for cystitis treatment recommend the use of antibiotics over 3–5 days. If the response is not satisfactory after 2–3 days after the start of the therapy, a change of the antibiotic should be considered based on the antibiogram [1, 22, 23, 26, 36].

Symptomatic therapy should include hydration, and in cases of pronounced dysuria, analgetics should be considered [11, 37].

The use of **antibiotic prophylaxis** over the decades in children with recurrent and complicated urinary tract infections is believed to have contributed to the preservation of kidney function in many patients. Its true benefit is nowadays a matter of debate, as well as the contribution of such a prophylactic use of antibiotics to the development of increasing antibiotic resistance [36, 38]. Analyzing numerous studies dealing with this issue, a consensus has been reached for patients with high-grade VUR (III–V) and repeated UTIs (three and more over a year). Another group of patients at risk and deserving of prophylactic use of antibiotics are patients with dysfunctional voiding and secondary VUR [22, 39]. The antibiotic of choice should be nitrofurantoin, although there are studies on the prophylactic use of cefaclor and trimethoprim-sulfamethoxazole [22, 32]. One should keep in mind the growing resistance of proteus to nitrofurantoin [40]. The dosage should be 1/3 of the therapeutic dose of the chosen antibiotic. The duration of prophylactic use should be individually determined [23, 26].

In cases of fungal urinary tract infection, systemic antimycotic therapy is indicated. Asymptomatic fungal cystitis in otherwise healthy children does not need any treatment. In cases of fungal infection in neonates, infants, and immunocompromised children, as well as before invasive urological procedures antimycotic therapy is recommended for the prevention of systemic infection. Symptomatic cystitis treatment with fluconazole as an antimycotic of choice is recommended for two weeks, or in cases where fluconazole is not an option, same length of treatment with amphotericin B. There are some data on intravesical irrigation of the bladder with amphotericin B (500 mg/1 l of saline). However, there is a lack of sufficient randomized studies with clear treatment recommendations in this regard. Irrigation of the bladder in fungal cystitis should be considered in patients with refractory fungal cystitis with strains resistant to conventional antimycotic medications. In cases of urinary obstruction with "fungus ball," surgical intervention is indicated [12, 41].

Viral cystitis in most cases resolves on its own. Complete regression of the symptoms happens after 2–3 weeks. Symptomatic therapy is usually sufficient. Lately, the use of cidofovir is discussed in infection with polyoma BK and Adenovirus. Due to its high level of nephrotoxicity, its use is still debatable, and further studies are necessary [2, 42].

Contemporary guidelines do not recommend treatment of asymptomatic bacteriuria, except before invasive surgical procedures (**Tables 2** and **3**) [11, 22, 43].

Medications	Dosage	Comment
Amoxicillin/clavulanic acid	20–50 mg/kg/day divided q8h	Based on amoxicillin component
Cephalexin	25–50 mg/kg/day divided q8h	/
Cefixime	8 mg/kg/day q24h	Age < 6 months safety and efficacy not established
Cefpodoxime	10 mg/kg/day divided q12h	Age < 1 months safety and efficacy not established
Cefuroxime	30 mg/kg/day divided q12h	Age < 3 months safety and efficacy not established
Nitrofurantoin	5–7 mg/kg divided q6h	Nitrofurantoin is not suitable for the treatment of cystitis + pyelonephritis, because of its limited tissue penetration.
Trimethoprim—sulfamethoxazole (TMP-SMZ)	8 mg/kg/day, divided q12h	Based on TMP component. Contraindicated in hyperbilirubinemia and age < 1 months

Prophylactic dosage should be 1/3 of the therapeutic dose of the chosen antibiotic.
If it is needed, adjust dose in renal insufficiency.

Table 2.
Antibiotic agents for the oral treatment and prophylactic options of cystitis.

Medications	Dosage and route	Comment
Ceftriaxone	50–75 mg/kg/day IV/IM as a single dose or divided q12h	Do not use in infants age < 6 weeks may displace bilirubin from albumin
Cefotaxime	150 mg/kg/day IV/IM divided q6-8h	Safe to use in infants age < 6 weeks
Amoxicillin/clavulanic acid	100–150 mg/kg/day IV divided q6-8h	Indicated for complicated UTIs approved from birth and older
Amikacin	15 mg/kg/day IV/IM in single dose or divided q12h	/
Gentamicin	7.5 mg/kg/dose/day IV divided q8h	/

For neonates and preterms consult neonatal antimicrobial guidelines.
If it is needed, adjust dose in renal insufficiency.

Table 3.
Antibiotic agents for parenteral treatment of cystitis.

9. Imaging after UTI

Imaging after UTI is needed to rule out an underlying renal or urinary tract anomaly or the assessment of a renal injury.

Renal ultrasound is a useful diagnostic tool for evaluating urinary tract anomalies, urinary obstruction, renal structural anomalies, nephrolithiasis, calcification or an abdominal mass. In the last decade, the practice patterns have dramatically shifted, with far fewer patients undergoing voiding cystourethrogram (VCUG) after an initial UTI [1, 3]. Nevertheless, in children with abnormal ultrasound, atypical causative pathogen, complex clinical course or known renal scarring, and voiding cystourethrography should be considered to exclude vesicoureteral reflux [2].

DMSA scan is considered as the current gold standard for the assessment of renal parenchymal injury in children with a history of febrile UTI. However, most children with first febrile UTI do not need a DMSA renal scan [27]. It may be considered in children with recurrent febrile UTIs or renal parenchymal abnormalities on ultrasound [3]. Findings of renal scarring may influence surgical decision making in patients with surgically correctable conditions such as VUR. Renal scars on DMSA scans performed during or shortly after acute pyelonephritis may be due to preexisting acquired or congenital lesions or to the acute inflammatory reaction associated with APN. It is therefore recommended to perform a delayed DMSA scan at 4 to 6 months. A delayed scan allows the acute inflammatory reaction to subside, at which point any persistent cortical defects can be considered as renal scars, although in the absence of baseline scans, it may still be difficult to differentiate acquired from congenital lesions [3].

10. Prevention

Repeated cystitis is usually correlated with VUR, urolithiasis, or bowel and bladder elimination syndrome. All of those patients should be offered urotherapy, consisting of timed voiding (every 3 h), double micturition (to avoid residual urine), and other behavioral changes, including avoidance of urine withholding behavior in toilet-trained children. Specific management of obstipation should be offered for the patient. Biofeedback might be offered for patients with bowel and bladder elimination syndrome. In children with urolithiasis, the basis for the prevention of urinary infection is the management of the specific metabolic cause of urolithiasis, through dietary and medicamentous therapy. A very important factor in the prevention of urinary tract infections is adequate hydration [11, 44–46].

Antibiotics can harm gastrointestinal and periurethral flora, compromising in such a way the host's defense mechanisms against pathogenic bacteria. The critical use of antibiotics in treating infections or other diseases is mandatory [3].

It has been scientifically proven that circumcision is beneficial in reducing the incidence of urinary infections in certain boys. Routine circumcision is, however, not recommended [19, 22].

The use of probiotics prevents colonization of the bowel with pathogenic bacteria with regular hygienic measures involving the prepuce and perineum. Their use is, however, not correlated with a significantly reduced incidence of recurrent UTIs [11, 47].

The prophylactic effects of cranberries have not been well documented. Some studies have shown that regular use of cranberry juice (minimum 6 months) reduces the number of repeated cystitis in children [48].

11. Complications

Usually, acute complication of cystitis includes dehydration, electrolyte disturbances, and febrile seizures. Intravenous hydration is necessary in more severe cases, often in younger children. Also, the use of some nephrotoxic drugs, such as non-steroidal anti-inflammatory drugs and antibiotics, can lead to acute kidney injury [3, 49]. Severe blood loss as a consequence of hemorrhagic cystitis caused by chemotherapeutics is very rare but a significant factor affecting the morbidity and mortality in pediatric oncologic patients [2, 11].

If cystitis is not timely diagnosed and adequately treated, it can progress into pyelonephritis, carrying the risk of kidney scars and loss of kidney function in the future. Also, in the case of repeated cystitis with associated VUR or bladder dysfunction, there is a greater chance of renal scarring. In most children, renal scarring may not be clinically significant, but it may cause hypertension, proteinuria, and progressive decline in renal function as long-term complication of cystitis and UTI in general [49, 50].

Cystitis in the pediatric population in addition to being a health problem also has a great socioeconomic significance. Considering their frequency, tendency for recurrence, as well as the sequelae that can develop in the future, they have consequences not only for individual, but also for whole society.

12. Conclusion

Cystitis in children is usually a mild disease with a good prognosis. Nevertheless, due to specific conditions sometimes associated with cystitis in pediatric population (VUR, DSD...), it requires careful patient evaluation, adequate diagnostic procedures, and treatment. It is a common condition that is often undiagnosed and should not be underestimated.

Author details

Dragana Živković[1,2]* and Maja Samardžić Lukić[1,2]

1 Faculty of Medicine, University of Novi Sad, Serbia

2 Institute for Child and Youth Health Care of Vojvodna, Novi Sad, Serbia

*Address all correspondence to: zivkica974@gmail.com

References

[1] 't Hoen LA, Bogaert G, Radmayr C, Dogan HS, et al. Update of the EAU/ESPU guidelines on urinary tract infections in children. Journal of Pediatric Urology. 2021;**17**:200-207

[2] Goldberg B, Jantausch B. Urinary tract infection. In: Kher KK, Schnaper WH, Greenbaum LA, editors. Clinical Pediatric Nephrology. 3rd ed. New York: CRC Press; 2020. pp. 967-991

[3] Matoo TK, Shaikh N. Contemporary Management of Urinary Tract Infection in children. Pediatrics. 2021;**147**(2):e2020012138

[4] Rc P, Popescu RI, Toma C, Dumitrascu MC, et al. Chemical hemorrhagic cystitis: Diagnostic and therapeutic pitfalls (review). Experimental and Therapeutic Medicine. 2021;**21**:624

[5] Stein R, Dogan HS, Hoebeke P, Kočvara R, et al. Urinary tract infections in children: EAU/ASPU Giudelines. European Urology. 2015;**67**(3):546-558

[6] van der Voort J, Edwards A, Roberts R, Verrier JK. The struggle to diagnose UTI in children under two in primary care. Family Practice. 1997;**14**:44-48

[7] Ladomenou F, Bitsori M, Galanakis E. Incidence and morbidity of urinary tract infection in a prospective cohort of children. Acta pediatrica. International Journal of Pediatrics. 2015;**104**(7):e324-e329

[8] Boon H, Strufyf T, Crevecoeur J, Delvaux J, et al. Incidence rates and trends of childhood urinary tract infections and antibiotic prescribing. Registry-based study in general practice (2000-2020). BMC Primary Care. 2022;**23**:177

[9] Tullus K, Shaikh N. Urinary tract infections in children. Lancet. 2020;**395**:1659-1668

[10] Schlager TA. Urinary tract infections in infants and children. Microbiol Spectrum. 2016;**4**(5):UTI-0022-2016

[11] Rees L, Bockenhauer D, Webb N, Punaro MG. Oxford Specialist Handbooks in Pediatrics Pediatric Nephrology. 3rd ed. New York: Oxford University Press, Oxford University Press; 2019. pp. 87-102

[12] Murillo JL, Lee WM, Al Sheikh S, Tulsyan V, Cohen M. Amfotericin B bladder irrigation for the treatment of neonatal bladder fungus ball. Journal of Pediatric Infectious Diseases. 2012;**4**(7):165-169

[13] Gorczynska E, Turkiewicz D, Rybka K, et al. Incidence, clinical outcomeand management of virus-induced hemorrhagic cystitis in children and adolescens after allogenic hematopoetic cell transplantation. Biology of Blood and Marrow Transplantation. 2005;**11**:797-804

[14] Robinson D, Schulz G, Langley R, Donze K, Winchester K, Rodgers C. Evidence-based practice recommendations for hydration in children and adolescents with cancer receiving intravenous cyclophosphamide. Journal of Pediatric Oncology Nursing. 2017;**31**(4):191-199

[15] Thompson A, Adamson A, Bahl A, Borwell J, et al. Guidelines for the diagnosis, prevention and management of chemical- and radiation-induced

cystitis. Journal of Clinical Urology. 2014;**7**:25-35

[16] Simoes e Silva AC, Oliveira EA, Mak RH. Urinary tract infection in pediatrics: An overview. Jornal de Pediatria. 2020;**96**(s1):65-79

[17] Ballek NK, McKenna PH. Lower urinary tract dysfunction in childhood. The Urologic Clinics of North America. 2010;**37**:215-228

[18] Hooton TM, Scholes D, Hughes JP, et al. A prospective study of risk factors for symptomatic urinary tract infection in young women. The New England Journal of Medicine. 1996;**335**:468

[19] Singh-Grewal D, Macdessi J, Craig J. Circumsicion for the prevention of urinary tract infection in boys: A sistem review of randomised trials and observational studies. Archives of Disease in Childhood. 2005;**90**:853-858

[20] Ambite I, Rydstrom G, Schwaderer AL, Hains DS. The genetics of urinary tract infections and the innate Defense of the kidney and urinary tract. Journal of Pediatric Genetics. 2016;**5**:25-32

[21] Zaffanello M, Melrba G, Cataldi L, Antoniazzi F, et al. Genetic risk for recurrent urinary tract infections in humans: A systemic review. Journal of Biomedicine & Biotechnology. 2010;**2010**:321082

[22] European Association of Urology. Guidelines on Paediatric Urology. 2022 [internet publication]

[23] Buettcher M, Trueck J, Niederer-Loher A, Heininger U, et al. Swiss consensus recommendations on urinary tract infections in children. European Journal of Pediatrics. 2021;**180**:663-674

[24] Shaikh N, Borell JL, Evron J, MMG L. Procalcitonin, C reactive protein and erythrocyte sedimentation rate for the diagnosis of acute pyelonephritis in children. Cochrane Database of Systematic Reviews. 2015;**1**:CD009185

[25] Leroy S, Gervaix A. Procalcitonin, a useful biomarker in pediatric urinary tract infection. Archives de Pédiatrie. 2013;**20**:50-64

[26] Ammenti A, Alberici I, Brugnara M, Chimenz R. Update Italian recommendations for the diagnosis, treatment and follow-up of the first febrile urinary tract infection in young children. Acta Pediatrica. 2020;**109**:236-247

[27] Subcommittee on urinary tract infection; steering committee on quality improvement and management. Urinary tract infection: Clinical practice guideline for the diagnosis and Management of the Initial UTI in febrile infants and children 2 to 24 months. Pediatrics. Sep 2011;**128**(3):595-610

[28] Diviney J, Jaswon MS. Urine collection methods and dipstick testing in non-toilet-trained children. Pediatric Nephrology. 2021;**36**:1697-1708

[29] Labrosse M, Levy A, Autmizguine J, Gravel J. Evaluation of a new strategy for clean-catch urine in infants. Pediatrics. 2016;**138**:e20160573

[30] Kaufman J, Fitzpatrick P, Tosif S, et al. Faster clean catch urine collection (quick-wee method) from infants: Randomized controlled trial. BMJ. 7 Apr 2017;**357**:j1341-1348

[31] Tullus K. Defining urinary tract infection by bacterial colony counts: A case for less than 100,000 colonies/mL as the threshold. Pediatric Nephrology. 2019;**34**:1651-1653

[32] Uwaezuoke S, Ayuk A, Muoneke U. Urinary tract infection in

children: A review of the established practice guidelines. European Journal of Clinical Microbiology & Infectious Diseases. 2020;**1**(1):57-65

[33] Duffy MA, Hernandez Santigo V, Orange G, Davey PG, Guthrie B. Trimethoprim prescription and subsequent resistance in childhood urinary infection: Multilevel modeling analysis. The British Journal of General Practice. 2013;**22**:1133-1137

[34] European Medicines Agency. Disabling and potentially permanent side effects lead to suspension or restrictions of quinolone and fluoroquinolone antibiotics. EMA. 2018:795349

[35] Gokce I, Çicek N, Guven S, et al. Changes in bacterial resistance patterns of pediatric urinary tract infections and rationale for empirical antibiotic therapy. Balkan Medical Journal. 2017;**34**:432-435

[36] Robinson JL, Le Saux N. Management of urinary tract infections in children in an era of increasing antimicrobial resistance. Expert Review of Anti-Infective Therapy. 2016;**14**:809-816

[37] Fasugba O, Mitchell BG, McInnes E, et al. Increased fluid intake for the prevention of urinary tract infection in adults and children in all settings: A systematic review. The Journal of Hospital Infection. 2020;**104**(1):68-77

[38] Selekman RE, Shapiro DJ, Boscardin J, Williams G, et al. Uropathogen resistance and antibiotic prophylaxis: A meta-analysis. Pediatrics. 2018;**142**:e20180119

[39] The RIVUR Trial Investigators. Antimicrobial prophylaxis for children with vesicoureteral reflux. The New England Journal of Medicine. 2014;**370**:2367-2376

[40] Huttner A, Verhaegh EM, Harbarth S, Muller AE, Theuretzbacher U, Mouton JW. Nitrofurantoin revisited: A systematic review and meta-analysis of controlled trials. The Journal of Antimicrobial Chemotherapy. 2015;**70**:2456-2464

[41] Pappas PG, Ca K, Andes D, et al. Clinical practice guidelines for the management of candidiasis: 2009 update by the Infectious Diseases Society of America. Clinical Infectious Diseases. 2009;**48**:503-535

[42] Yusuf U, Hale GA, Carr J, et al. Cidofovir for the treatment of adenoviral infection in pediatric hematopoietic stem cell transplat patients. Transplantion. 2006;**81**:1398-1404

[43] Nicolle LE. Asymptomatic bacteriuria. Current Opinion in Infectious Diseases. 2014;**27**:90-96

[44] Shaikh N, Hoberman A, Keren R, Gotman N, et al. Recurrent urinary tract infections in children with bladder and bowel dysfunction. Pediatrics. 2016;**137**:e20152982

[45] Hoebeke P, Bower W, Combs A, de Jong T, Yang S. Diagnostic evaluation of children with daytime incontinence. The Journal of Urology. 2010;**183**:699-703

[46] Panzarino V. Urolithiasis in children. Advances in Pediatrics. 2020;**67**:105-112

[47] Schwenger EM, Tejani AM, Loewen PS. Probiotics for preventing urinary tract infections in children and adults. Cochrane Database of Systematic Reviews. 23 Dec 2015;**2015**(12)

[48] Salo J, Uhari M, Helminen M, et al. Cranberry juice for the prevention of recurrences of urinary tract infections in children: A randomized

placebo-controlled trial. Clinical Infectious Diseases. 2012;**54**:340-346

[49] Roberts KB. Urinary tract infections and renal damage: Focusing on what matters. JAMA Pediatrics. 2014;**168**(10):884-885

[50] Salo J, Ikaheimo R, Tapiainen T, Uhari M. Childhood urinary tract infections as cause of chronic kidney disease. Pediatrics. 2011;**128**(5):840-847

Chapter 4

Interstitial Cystitis/Bladder Pain Syndrome

Asad Ullah and Muhammad Jamil

Abstract

Interstitial cystitis/bladder pain syndrome (IC/BPS) is a heterogeneous, chronic, and debilitating condition. It affects 400,000 individuals in the United Kingdom. IC/BPS presents with suprapubic pain or discomfort perceived to be related to the urinary bladder with one or more urinary symptoms (e.g., urgency, frequency or nocturia) for more than 6 weeks. The exact etiology is not clearly understood. It can sometimes co-exist with other chronic pain disorders, complicating the diagnosis and management. IC/BPS can adversely impact the quality of life, impede work, and interfere with the sleep, sexual and social life of the affected individual. The contemporary treatments are palliative and aim for symptom control only. There is no cure available presently. Moreover, treatment effects are highly variable; therefore, personalization of treatment is vital for achieving the desired outcomes. Management includes lifestyle modifications, physical therapy, systemic pharmacotherapy, intravesical therapies and surgery. Conservative treatments are usually used first, followed by invasive and combination therapies if required. Treatment should aim beyond symptom improvement and encompass improvement in quality of life. Further research is needed to understand the etiology and pathophysiology of IC/BPS. It will assist in the development of new biomarkers and drug development.

Keywords: bladder pain, chronic pelvic pain, interstitial cystitis/bladder pain syndrome, Hunner lesion, intravesical therapies

1. Introduction

Interstitial cystitis or bladder pain syndrome (IC/BPS) is a chronic debilitating condition of uncertain etiology. The American Urology Association (AUA) guidelines define IC/BPS as 'an unpleasant sensation (pain, pressure, discomfort) perceived to be related to the urinary bladder, associated with lower urinary tract symptoms of more than 6 weeks duration in the absence of infection or other identifiable causes.' [1].

The exact etiology of IC/BPS is unknown. Most of the affected patients have a poor quality of life. It is a diagnosis of exclusion, meaning that IC/BPS is diagnosed when other conditions causing similar symptoms are excluded. IC/BPS may coexist with other painful conditions, such as irritable bowel syndrome, fibromyalgia etc., which can delay the diagnosis and complicate management. No cure is available yet, and the existing therapies target symptom control and palliation. No treatment has shown a clinically meaningful advantage over the other.

Moreover, the available treatments are not equally effective in all patients. Therefore, it is essential to tailor the management according to the patient's needs. Management of IC/BPS is best delivered in a multidisciplinary approach and should focus on the quality of life in addition to symptoms.

2. Nomenclature and classification

The term interstitial cystitis is misleading. The symptoms of interstitial cystitis are not reliably associated with the pathology of bladder interstitium. Moreover, bladder inflammation (cystitis) is not observed in all cases of IC/BPS. The term IC was changed to painful bladder syndrome and later replaced by bladder pain syndrome. In the Japanese and East Asian literature, 'hypersensitive bladder' is used for IC/BPS, further complicating the nomenclature. The terminology of IC/BPS needs standardization for clarity.

For historical reasons, IC/BPS are reported together. In this chapter, the term IC/BPS will be used.

3. Epidemiology

The exact incidence and prevalence of IC/BPS are unknown due to the lack of formalized diagnostic criteria. It is frequently reported in middle-aged men (55-75 yr) and women (50-60 yr). IC/BPS predominately affects females (female: male ratio 10:1). The prevalence of self-reported disease ranges from 850 per 100,000 in women and 60 per 100,000 in men [2, 3]. Based on this data, approximately 1.2 million women and 83,000 men have IC/BPS in the United States. Medical billing-based prevalence of IC/BPS is slightly lower, 197 per 100,000 in women and 41 per 100,000 in men [3]. The prevalence of IC/BPS in Europe is low (8-16 per 100,000) [4]. IC/BPS prevalence is believed to be very low in children.

4. Etiology and pathophysiology

The etiology of IC/BPS is not fully understood. Some of the proposed theories are mentioned below. However, none of these theories has been proven.

- Good concordance of IC/BPS in monozygotic twins suggests genetic vulnerability [5].

- Urinary tract infection- bacterial or viral infection in the bladder induces an inflammatory process which continues even after clearing the infection.

- Leaky Glycosaminoglycan (GAG) layer- bladder urothelium is covered by glycosaminoglycans (GAG) which act as a protective lining against bacteria and irritants in the urine. It is hypothesized that disruption of the GAG layer results in increased permeability. Irritants in the urine, such as Potassium, depolarize the muscles and nerves in the bladder wall. It, in turn, triggers inflammation and degranulation of mast cells causing lower urinary tract symptoms.

- Autoimmune reaction- autoimmunity may sometimes be responsible for IC/BPS.

- Hypersensitivity reaction- In some cases, mast cell proliferation in the bladder wall biopsies is observed. They release histamines which cause hypersensitivity reactions, thus contributing to the IC/BPS symptoms.

- A functional brain magnetic resonance imaging (MRI) study of patients with IC/BPS revealed an increase in the gray matter volume in brain areas related to pain [6], highlighting the role of the nervous system in the disease.

- Neurologic upregulation- some experts believe that recurrent bladder wall inflammation or irritation results in hyperplasia of the sensory nerves, enhancing pain perception. Repeated painful stimuli also induce changes in the spinal neurons making the signals robust and long-lasting.

- Recreational use of ketamine is associated with severe IC/BPS. Possible explanations include autoimmunity, infection, urothelial damage, and vascular changes due to ketamine or metabolites. Interestingly, ketamine use within the approved doses is not associated with bladder symptoms [7].

5. Clinical features

Pain exacerbated by bladder filling is the trademark of IC/BPS. Bladder pain is accompanied by one or more lower urinary tract symptoms such as urgency, urinary frequency and nocturia. Some patients complain of discomfort, pressure, or spasms in the suprapubic area instead of pain. The emergence of lower urinary tract symptoms may precede pain in some cases. Urgency is a notable symptom of an overactive bladder. However, the quality of urgency differs from IC/BPS. Patients with overactive bladder void to avert incontinence, while those with IC/BPS void to alleviate the pain. Some patients may experience extra bladder pain, e.g., in the lower abdomen, back, urethra, rectum, vulva, and vagina.

Urinary incontinence is uncommon in IC/PBS. In men, the symptoms of chronic prostatitis overlap with IC/BPS and need expert input to differentiate the two.

The disease usually commences with few symptoms, which progress to multiple symptoms. Symptoms typically build gradually; however, some patients may present acutely. The severity of the symptoms varies. Aggravating factors include sexual intercourse, exercise, prolonged sitting, psychosocial stress, menstruation and with certain foods or drinks.

Hypertonic pelvic floor dysfunction is common in IC/BPS. It is likely due to sensitization of thoracolumbar and sacral nerves. Some patients will have allodynia.

Physical examination demonstrates tenderness in the suprapubic area, perineum, lower back, levator muscles, and genitalia.

IC/BPS frequently affects the patient's social, psychological, and emotional well-being [8]. Depression, anxiety, panic disorder, abnormal work-life balance and sexual dysfunction are more prevalent in IC/BPS than controls. IC/BPS patients complain of moderate to severe sexual dysfunction. Pain is the primary driver of sexual dysfunction.

Moreover, other chronic pain syndromes such as irritable bowel syndrome, fibromyalgia, chronic headaches, Sjogren's syndrome and vulvodynia may coexist with IC/BPS.

IC/BPS adversely impact on quality of life (QoL). It is associated with decreased work productivity, disturbed sleep, emotional changes, sexual dysfunction, and reduced mobility. The effects on QoL are as severe as reported in maintenance hemodialysis, rheumatoid arthritis, Crohn's disease, and systemic lupus erythematosus.

The clinical course of the disease is not fully understood. Some patients reported spontaneous resolution of symptoms, while other studies reported a waxing and waning course with a slight improvement over time [9, 10].

6. Diagnosis

IC/BPS is a diagnosis of exclusion. No definitive diagnostic test for IC/BPS exists apart from IC/BPS with Hunner lesion, diagnosed on cystoscopy. The diagnosis is delayed in most cases by 5-6 years [11]. Detailed history taking, examination and laboratory investigations help reach the diagnosis.

According to AUA 2022 guidelines, cystoscopy is not essential for diagnosing IC/BPS. However, cystoscopy is performed to exclude other differential diagnoses. IC/BPS with Hunner lesion is an exception where cystoscopy is diagnostic. Cystoscopy is also indicated in IC/BPS patients who fail to respond to initial treatment to exclude alternative diagnoses.

ICP/BPS with Hunner lesion was first described by Guy Leroy Hunner in 1914. Hunner lesion in the acute phase is a confined, erythematous mucosa with tiny blood vessels radiating toward the center of a pale scar [12] (**Figure 1**). A Fibrin clot is attached to the lesion. Hunner lesions may bleed after hydrodistension in a waterfall

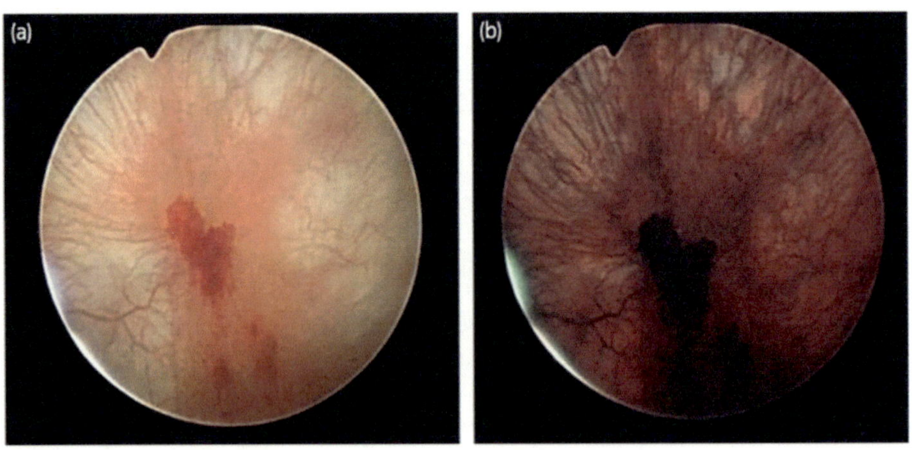

Figure 1.
A Hunner lesion. (a) Hunner lesion is a reddish muscosal lesion lacking the normal capillary structure, frequently covered by fibrin clots. (b) Narrow-band imaging cystoscopy of the Hunner lesion emphaizes the abnormal capillary structure converging toward the lesion (Reproduced with permission).

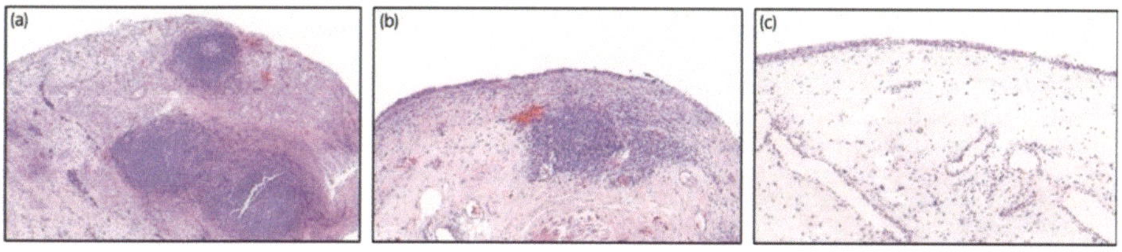

Figure 2.
Histological features of IC/BPS. (a) IC/BPS with Hunner lesions (lesion area). Dense subepithelial inflammatory infiltrates, epithelial denudation and increased neovascularization are observed, often accompanied by lymph follicles (magnification: x100). (b) IC/BPS with Humner lesion (non-lesion are). Note that similar inflammatory changes observed in a non-lesion area (magnification: x200). (c) IC/BPS without Hunner lesions. Few inflammatory changes with retained urothelium (magnification: x200) (Reproduced with permission).

pattern. Chronic lesions are blanched and do not bleed. Microscopy of the Hunner lesion shows chronic infiltrate consisting of neutrophils, eosinophils, lymphocytes, plasma cells, macrophages, and mast cells [12] (**Figure 2**).

Hunner lesions are found in only 5-10% of the cases. The multidisciplinary approach to pelvic pain (MAPP) phase II study revealed Hunner lesions in 19.7% between 50 and 70 and 54.5% over the age of 70 yr. [13]. Hunner lesions respond well to treatment. Therefore, it is appropriate to offer early cystoscopy in this age group.

Glomerulations or reactive petechial hemorrhages are observed in some cases. They are non-specific and non-diagnostic. They can be seen in other conditions, e.g., radiation cystitis, bladder cancer and sometimes in healthy individuals. Moreover, glomerulations do not correlate with symptoms of IC/BPS [14].

Urodynamic tests are non-specific and could cause discomfort. Therefore, they are not recommended routinely in diagnosing IC/BPS.

The Potassium sensitivity test (PST) informs about urothelial permeability and dysfunction [15]. It is non-specific and may be positive in urinary tract infection and radiation cystitis. It could be painful and might cause a severe flare-up. Furthermore, PST is not predictive of response to urothelium restoring therapies.

Improvement of symptoms during an anesthetic bladder challenge (which involves the instillation of an anesthetic cocktail) is no longer recommended as a diagnostic test.

Differential diagnoses include bladder/urethral cancer, genital cancers, benign pelvic conditions (e.g., uterine fibroid, pelvic organ prolapse etc.), infections in the pelvic area, chronic pelvic pain syndromes, intravesical pathology (e.g., stone, foreign body etc.), urethral diverticulum, disorders causing bladder outflow obstruction (e.g., enlarged prostate), neurologic disorders, diabetes mellitus, bowel diseases (e.g., inflammatory bowel disease, diverticular disease), trauma, and radiation etc.

7. Assessment tools

Several validated questionnaires are available. Some could assist in diagnosis, while others are used to track changes in the symptoms after an intervention. Some questionnaires assess the impact of IC/BPS on QoL. **Table 1** illustrates some of the commonly used validated instruments.

Questionnaire	Domains	Additional information
O'Leary Sant/Interstitial cystitis symptoms and problem indexes [16]	Urinary symptoms, pain, general health, QoL, Sexual health & relationship with menses	Self-administered, monitor changes in symptoms, not a screening test
University of Wisconsin interstitial cystitis inventory (WICI) [17]	Pelvic pain, pelvic discomfort, urine frequency, nocturia, Urgency, dysuria & sleep	Used to monitor changes in the symptoms
Medical outcomes study 36-item short-form health survey (SF-36) [18]	General health, physical function, vitality, body pain, mental health, social function & emotional health	Focused on QoL
Pelvic pain and urinary frequency patient symptom scale (PUF) [19]	Urine frequency, nocturia, pain, QoL & sexual function	Helps in distinguishing bladder pain from reproductive tract pain and is correlated with the Potassium sensitivity test
UPOINT [20]	Urinary, psychosocial, organ specific, infection, neurological/ systematic & tenderness	Focused on QoL, Guides in phenotyping the disease
Bladder symptoms impact scale (BSI-6) [21]	Energy level, interest in daily activity, mood, social life, self-worth & ability to perform home activities.	Focused on QoL
King's Health questionnaire [22]	Sleep, physical limitation, role limitation, symptom bother & emotions	Focused on QoL
Global response assessment (GRA)	Disease symptoms	Monitors change in symptoms before and after treatment, non-specific
Visual analogue score (VAS)	Pain	Monitors change in symptoms before and after treatment, non-specific

Table 1.
Validated questionnaires for IC/BPS.

8. Phenotyping

IC/BPS comes under the umbrella term of chronic pain syndrome (**Figure 3**). Earlier guidelines did not classify IC/BPS into phenotypes. However, there is growing consensus among experts that IC/BPS is not a single disease but a spectrum. Furthermore, various phenotypes respond to different therapies. The AUA and East Asian Association of Urologists updated guidelines endorses this concept. According to the AUA IC/BPS guidelines 2022, IC/BPS has three distinct phenotypes.

- Bladder-centric phenotype- includes patients with Hunner lesions and small bladder capacity. They improve with intravesical anesthetics. Some experts even propose that IC/BPS with Hunner lesion is an entirely different disease and should not be considered part of BPS.

- Pelvic floor phenotype- exhibits pelvic floor tenderness on physical examination. This subgroup benefits from physical therapy.

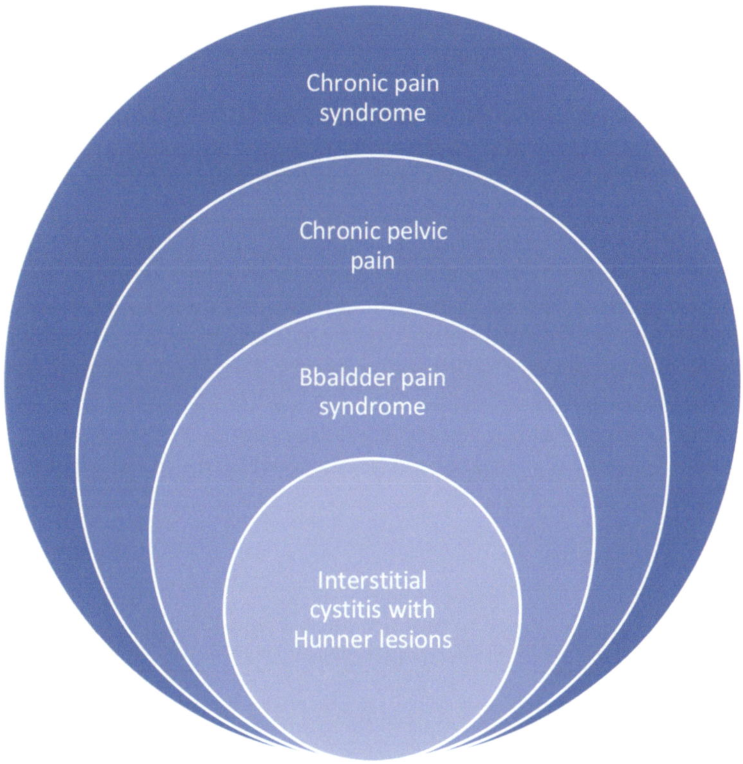

Figure 3.
Classification of IC/PBS.

- Systemic or widespread pain phenotype- has extra pelvic pain. These patients have chronic overlapping pain conditions (such as fibromyalgia, irritable bowel syndrome etc.), psychosocial issues and widespread somatic symptoms from multiple organs. These patients need a multidisciplinary treatment approach.

UPOINT (urinary, psychosocial, organ specific, infection, neurologic and or extra pelvic/systemic pain and tenderness of pelvic floor) phenotyping system is a valuable tool to characterize the different domains of the IC/BPS.

A study stratified IC/BPS patients using bladder capacity. Lower bladder capacity was associated with bladder-centric disease [23] with no associated somatic symptoms and affect dysregulation. Large bladder capacity was associated with extra bladder symptoms, e.g., functional somatic syndrome. They also had abnormal psychosocial history, e.g., childhood relationship problems, dissociative pathology etc. [24]. Further validation in extensive studies is warranted before recommending bladder capacity as a biomarker in IC/BPS.

Patients' stratification and phenotyping could assist in minimizing the variable response to the available treatments.

9. Treatment

Currently, there is no cure available for IC/BPS. The available treatments aim at the palliation of symptoms. Contemporary literature does not support one therapy over the other. It is, therefore, essential to personalize the treatment plans for each patient. Patients should be monitored after treatment; alternative therapies should replace ineffective treatments.

Realistic treatment goals should be outlined right at the inception. Patient-related outcomes should guide treatment goals. Every patient may not achieve the desired symptom control; therefore, the treatment should focus on minimizing the discomfort and improving the quality of life (**Figure 4**).

The earlier AUA guidelines (2014) recommended a hierarchal approach starting with conservative therapies first and progressing to invasive therapies. The latest AUA guidelines (2022) propose to design treatment plans based on patients' needs and risk-benefit assessment. Surgical treatments are not effective in every case and are associated with significant morbidity and mortality. Therefore, it should be used as a last resort in refractory disease.

Patients' education about the disease is vital to bring their expectations close to reality. Complex or resistant cases should be managed by multidisciplinary team approach (**Figure 5**).

9.1 Lifestyle modifications

Patients should be encouraged to practice lifestyle modification and self-care practices. A symptom diary could help in the identification of triggering or relieving factors.

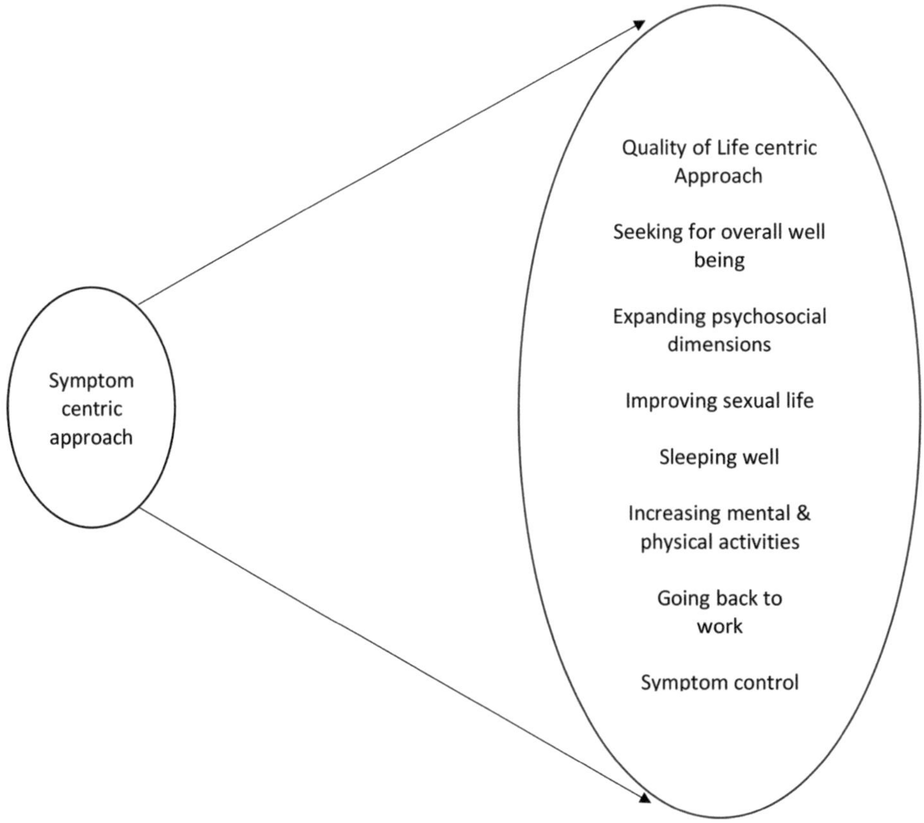

Figure 4.
Goals for managing IC/BPS.

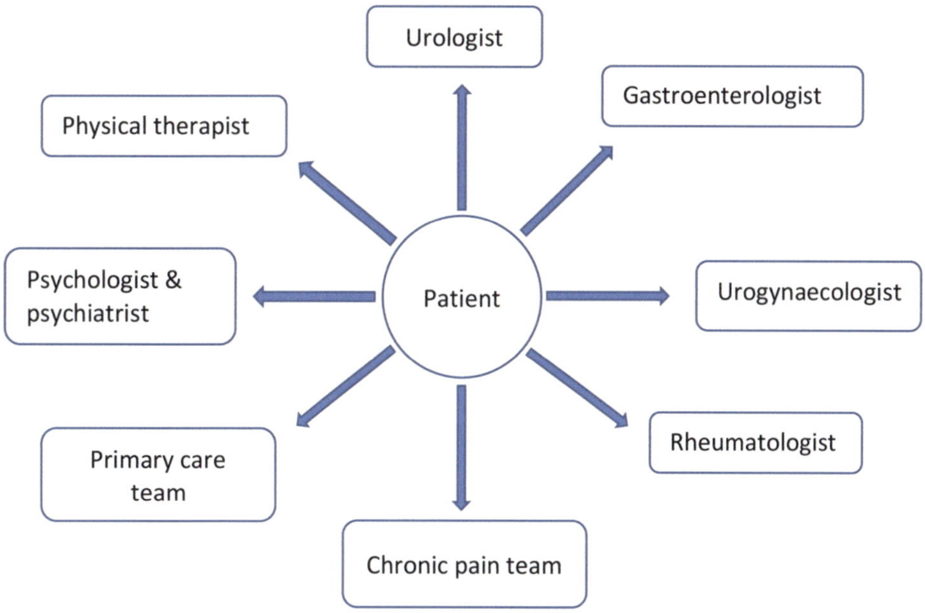

Figure 5.
Multidisciplinary team for managing IC/PBS.

Food characteristics [26]	Examples
Caffeine-containing food	Coffee, chocolate, tea, soda
Foods which make urine acidic	Citrus fruit, tomatoes, onions, Fava beans
Miscellaneous	Spicy foods, soya, alcoholic drinks, walnuts, pistachios, cashews, nut butter, processed meat or fish, rosemary, thyme, asparagus, broccoli, eggplant, spinach, water

Table 2.
Foods causing exacerbation of IC/BPS.

A moderate fluid restriction could improve bladder discomfort associated with filling. In contrast, those sensitive to concentrated urine may benefit from additional hydration.

More than 80% of patients describe sensitivity to food [25]. **Table 2** displays commonly reported culprit foods. Food sensitivity varies from patient to patient. A food diary and elimination diet could assist in spotting the culprit food or drinks.

Pelvic floor relaxation exercises such as squatting, reclining with spread legs, and placing knees against the chest wall can improve symptoms. These exercises increase void volume and interval between urination. Patients should avoid symptom aggravating activities, e.g., some types of physical exercises, recreational activities, and sexual activity. Kegel exercises which strengthen the pelvic floor are better avoided.

Cold or heat application over the bladder or perineum may comfort some patients. Timed voiding, bladder training to increase intervals between voids, and stress management strategies could be effective.

9.2 Physical therapy

Eighty-seven per cent of patients with IC/BPS have hypertonic pelvic floor muscle dysfunction [27]. It is unclear whether it is a primary pathology or a secondary phenomenon. Regardless of its origin, manual physical therapy can mitigate the symptoms.

Manual physical therapy focuses on releasing myofascial trigger points and is effective if palpation of the pelvis triggers the pain. Physical therapy delivered by an expert therapist renders good results.

A study randomly assigned 81 women with IC/BPS and pelvic floor tenderness to either pelvic floor myofascial physical therapy or full-body therapeutic massage. More patients in the physical therapy group experienced moderate to marked improvement in symptoms than in the therapeutic massage group (59 vs. 29%) [28]. The evidence about the role of other forms of massage therapies is scarce. Acupuncture may be effective, but the evidence is limited.

9.3 Pharmacotherapy

9.3.1 Oral pharmacotherapy

Amitriptyline is a tricyclic antidepressant. It blocks the reuptake of serotonin and noradrenaline. In addition, it has anticholinergic, beta3 agonist, sedative, antihistamine, and mast cell stabilization properties. Though not licensed, it is commonly used in IC/BPS. It is commenced at 10 mg and gradually titrated to 75-100 mg once daily. Clinical effects manifest in 4-6 weeks. A small, randomized study (n = 50) of IC/BPS cases compared amitriptyline with a placebo [29]. Sixty-three per cent of patients in the amitriptyline group reported improvement in O′ Leary Sant score compared to 4% in the placebo arm at 16 weeks. Another randomized study showed similar results in favor of amitriptyline (66 vs. 47%) [30]. Symptom control was better in patients who used 50 mg or a higher dose of amitriptyline (66 vs. 45%) at 3 months. Improvement in symptoms was insignificant when all amitriptyline doses were analyzed collectively (55 vs. 45%).

Toxicity (such as such as urinary retention, dry mouth, constipation, hypotension, weight gain, and dysrhythmia) limits the use of amitriptyline.

Amitriptyline is metabolized by cytochrome P450 (CYP450) enzymes. The risk of amitriptyline toxicity increases when co-adminstered with CYP450 inhibitors such as cimetidine, selective serotonin reuptake inhibitors and anticonvulsants. Concomitant use with monoamine oxidase inhibitors could result in Serotonin syndrome- a potentially life-threatening reaction. Amitriptyline can increase the arrhythmogenic effect of Cisapride.

Pentosan polysulphate sodium (PPS) (Elmron®) is a semi-synthetic polymer of xylose hydrogen sulphate. It can be administered orally or intravesical. PPS is the only United States Food and Drug Administration (FDA) approved oral drug for IC/BPS. Orally administered PPS is excreted in the urine restoring the damaged GAG layer over urothelium. The recommended oral dose is 100 mg three times a day. Clinical effects manifest in 3-6 months.

A meta-analysis showed improvement in frequency, urgency and pain with PPS compared to placebo [31]. However, recent RCTs demonstrate conflicting results, probably related to the study design. A RCT of 64 patients compared cyclosporin A (1.5 mg/kg) to PPS (100 mg TID). Cyclosporin A was more effective at all clinical outcomes than PPS (83 vs. 21%) [32]. Another RCT randomly assigned 368 patients either to PPS 100 mg OD, PPS 100 mg TID or placebo. It was terminated earlier due to futility [33]. A meta-analysis of six RCTs reported statistically significant improvement in urinary urgency, frequency, and bladder pain with PPS than placebo (12.4 vs. 9%) [34]. Another controlled trial (n = 41) showed benefits with concomitant use of low-dose heparin and PPS [35].

PPS is associated with diarrhea, nausea, reversible alopecia, and mild transaminitis. Pigmented retinopathy occurs in 16% of patients with long-term (at least 3 yr) use of oral PPS. It manifests as difficulty in reading, blurred vision, and slow adjustment to reduced light. Detailed ophthalmic history and retinal examination are recommended for those with preexisting eye problems. A regular retinal examination is advocated for all patients on PPS. The risk-benefit ratio of continuing PPS should be re-evaluated if pigmentary maculopathy occurs.

Some clinicians have used antihistamines based on the hypothesis that histamine released from mast cells in the bladder is sometimes responsible for IC/BPS. Hydroxyzine is an H1 blocker with anticholinergic activity. Studies have shown contradictory results. A RCT compared hydroxyzine alone or in combination with PPS to a placebo. The effect of hydroxyzine alone was like a placebo (23 vs. 13%). The combination of hydroxyzine + PPS had better efficacy than PPS alone (43 vs. 28%) [36]. Cimetidine is an H2 receptor blocker. It is associated with improvement in suprapubic pain and nocturia [37]. Further work is needed to justify its use in IC/BPS, especially in those with elevated mast cells on bladder biopsy.

Analgesics are usually used as an adjunct to other therapies, e.g., paracetamol or non-steroidal anti-inflammatory drugs (NSAIDs). Opioid analgesics could be considered, but long-term use is associated with dependency. Phenazopyridine and methenamine could be used alone or in conjunction with NSAIDs. Methenamine is contraindicated in patients with hepatic or renal impairment and gout. Phenazopyridine should be used only for 1-3 days due to the risk of methemoglobinemia and renal and hepatic dysfunction.

Neuropathic agents, e.g., gabapentin and pregabalin, sometimes show symptom improvement.

9.3.2 Intravesical pharmacotherapies

Intravesical therapies deliver the drug directly at the site of action, thus increasing bioavailability and reducing the risk of systemic exposure. These therapies could be used in acute flare-ups or as maintenance therapy. A variety of medications, often in combination, are used.

Dimethyl sulfoxide (DMSO) is one of the two intravesical drugs approved by the FDA for IC/BPS. It could be given alone but often used in combination with other drugs. The exact mechanism of action is unknown; however, it relaxes the bladder muscles, has anti-inflammatory properties, and stabilizes mast cells. DMSO is administered intravesical at 50 ml of 50%. The dose is repeated weekly for 6 weeks. If good results are achieved, another 6 weeks course could be prescribed, followed by a monthly dose.

A small RCT (n = 33) compared DMSO to saline placebo. Patients treated with DMSO reported improvement in subjective symptom scores (53 vs. 18%) as well as in urodynamic parameters and voiding diary (93 vs. 35%) [38]. Another study used a cocktail of DMSO, hydrocortisone, bupivacaine, and heparin in 55 women with IC/BPS [39]. At 5 yr. follow-up, 23-47% of patients reported significant improvement in O'Leary Sant symptom index and pain scores. One-third of the cases were in remission without the need for further treatment. Twenty-one per cent of women required oral medication for symptom control. Small bladder capacity (<500 ml), high urine frequency (≥ 15/day) and nocturia were predictors of poor response. Another RCT compared DMSO to intravesical 2% chondroitin sulphate weekly for 6 weeks in 36 patients [40]. More than 50% of patients in the DMSO group withdraw due to instillation associate pain, garlic smell and lack of efficacy. The dropout rate was only 27% in the chondroitin sulphate group. Chondroitin sulphate was more effective in symptom control (72.7 vs. 14%), nocturia (−2.4 vs. −0.7) and pain (−1.2 vs. −0.6). Due to insufficient convincing evidence, DMSO is unlicensed in some countries, e.g., the UK.

Intravesical heparin improves IC/BPS symptoms in some cases. An observational study instilled heparin weekly into the bladder for 3 months and followed patients for 6 months. The responders increased from 33% at week 1 to 90% at week 16; however, the beneficial effect declined to 16.7% at 6 months [41]. A randomized controlled trial showed efficacy in the short term when used with sodium bicarbonate or local anesthetic agents, e.g., lidocaine. A combination of intravesical heparin and alkalinized lidocaine relieved pain and urine urgency (50 vs. 13%) at 12 hours compared to a placebo [42]. Heparin does appear to have beneficial effects, but further research is required.

Intravesical Hyaluronic acid (HA) and Chondroitin sulfate (CS) repair the damaged GAGs layer. Observational studies show a 66-87% efficacy rate of intravesical HA. In a prospective study, 121 women with IC/BPS received 40 mg intravesical HA weekly. All the participants had positive potassium tests suggestive of damaged GAGs layer. Eighty-five per cent of patients reported symptom improvement [43]. Another study randomly assigned 42 patients to intravesical HA or CS. Pain scores improved significantly in both treatment arms at 6 months; however, the CS group showed more remarkable improvement in urinary frequency, nocturia and VAS pain score [44].

A combination of HA and CS was effective in some trials. It is as effective as DMSO but with a better side effect profile. A meta-analysis of 10 studies shows significant improvement in O'Leary-Sant and VAS scores with intravesical HA and a combination of HA + CS [45]. Adequately powered randomized trials are required to assess the role of HA alone and combination HA/CS therapy in IC/BPS.

A meta-analysis of intravesical therapies reported similar response rates for HA, CS and PPS [46].

Local anesthetic agents (1-2% lidocaine) provide immediate symptom relief in acute flare-ups. A RCT compared daily alkalinized lidocaine to placebo for 5 days. A significant proportion of patients in the lidocaine arm showed symptom improvement (30 vs. 24%) [47]. The benefit was substantial on day three but not on day 10.

Intravesical 'cocktails' are widely used in clinics, especially for acute flare-ups. Different combinations of steroids, GAGs layer treatments, anesthetic agents, and antibiotics constitute these cocktails. The evidence for their use is limited.

9.4 Vesical procedures

9.4.1 Bladder hydrodistention

Is performed under spinal or general anesthesia. It is assumed to work by disrupting the sensory nerves in the bladder wall [48]. Observational studies report short-term (3-6 months) benefits. Some experts believe repeated distention might result in bladder wall fibrosis and worsening of the symptoms. However, studies have not confirmed this effect.

There is no standard protocol for bladder distention. Distending the bladder with water to a distention pressure of 60-80 cm H_2O for approximately ≤10 min is typical. Side effects include worsening of symptoms in some cases (9%), bladder wall necrosis and rupture. Due to a lack of confirmatory evidence, the European Association of Urology does not recommend bladder hydrodistention.

9.4.2 Treating Hunner lesions

Are treated with fulguration, resection, laser coagulation ± triamcinolone injection. One hundred and three patients who underwent transurethral resection of Hunner lesion reported symptom relief in 89% of cases. Forty per cent of patients did not require further treatment for 3 yrs.; however, the remaining 60% of cases needed repeated treatments (2-4 resections) [49]. The outcomes of resection are like fulguration.

Triamcinolone injection into the lesion improves symptoms in 70-74% of cases. The beneficial effects last for up to 12 months [50]. A systematic review of 13 studies using different procedures reported improvement in symptoms and quality of life; however, recurrence was reported [51].

A study used laser ablation (Neodymium: yttrium aluminum garnet) in 24 patients with Hunner lesions. All study participants reported reduced urgency, pain scores and nocturia [52]. The time between the void increased from 30 minutes to 100 minutes. The disease relapsed in 46% of cases but achieved good results with repeat ablation. Ablation is less invasive than resection or coagulation. Therefore, will cause minmal fibrosis. However, it needs confirmation.

9.5 Miscellaneous therapies

None of the following therapies is approved for IC/BPS; however, benefits are reported in refractory cases. It is essential to inform patients about the side effects. Experienced healthcare providers should administer these therapies.

Botulinum toxin A (BTX-A) injection into detrusor muscles improves IC/BPS symptoms by inhibiting muscle contractions, sensory nerves modulation and anti-inflammatory effects. A randomized controlled trial compared two doses of intra-detrusor BTX-A injection (200 and 100 units) + bladder hydrodistention and hydrodistention alone. BTX-A group reported moderate to a marked improvement in symptoms compared to hydrodistension alone (80 vs. 72 vs. 48% at 3 months). The benefits declined in all the groups at 24 months but more so in the hydrodistention alone group [53]. The 200 units of BTX-A did not add much to the efficacy but was associated with more adverse events. A third of the cases in the 200 units BTX-A group experienced urinary retention. Other studies have reported similar results. The patient should be informed about the possibility of clean intermittent self-catheterization.

Cyclosporine A is a calcineurin inhibitor. It modulates T cells and is an immunosuppressant agent. It is associated with significant toxicity, such as hypertension, nephrotoxicity, increased risk of infections, and malignancy. It is, therefore, reserved for those who failed the less toxic therapeutic options.

Studies show that cyclosporine A is particularly effective in IC/BPS with Hunner lesions compared to non-Hunner lesion phenotypes [54–56]. A study randomly assigned 64 patients to either cyclosporine A (1.5 mg/Kg BID) or PPS (100 mg TID) for 6 months [32]. Patients in the cyclosporine group showed more remarkable improvement on the symptom scale (75 vs. 19%) and in urinary frequency (−6.7 vs. −2.0 times per day). However, 94% of the patients in the cyclosporine A arm reported side effects.

Sacral neuromodulation (SNM) has shown variable results. SNM targets the sacral or pudendal nerve. Studies have reported preferential improvement in urinary frequency and urgency but not pain. A cross-over RCT prospectively compared sacral to pudendal nerve stimulation in 22 patients with refractory IC/BPS. Each patient used temporary sacral and pudendal nerve modulation separately. More patients opted for pudendal nerve stimulation. At 6 months, 59% of patients with pudendal nerve stimulation reported improved overall symptoms compared to 44% with sacral nerve stimulation [57]. Long-term follow-up data are lacking. It may be helpful in selected patients. Transcutaneous electrical nerve stimulation (TENS) and percutaneous tibial nerve stimulation (PTNS) have shown efficacy in small studies in selected patients.

Long-term use of antibiotics and steroids is not recommended anymore. Furthermore, intravesical instillation of bacillus Calmette-Guerin is no longer advised except in research studies. The efficacy of high-pressure and longer-duration hydrodistention is unpredictable and associated with complications. Therefore, it should not be offered.

9.6 Surgery

Surgery is the last resort option in patients who fail all other therapies but still have significant symptoms. It is associated with considerable morbidity and mortality. Furthermore, every patient may not benefit from surgery. Therefore, patient selection is of utmost importance for achieving the desired outcomes. Limited data suggest that patients with Hunner lesions, small bladder capacity under anesthesia and fibrotic bladder respond to surgery. Those with an extra bladder source of pain are unlikely to benefit from bladder surgery.

The purpose of surgery is to increase bladder capacity or to divert urine from the bladder. The selection of the operative technique depends on the patient and surgeon-specific factors. The options include bladder augmentation cystoplasty, cystoplasty with or without supra-trigone resection, and urinary diversion with or without cystectomy. Each procedure has its unique advantages and complications.

A systematic review of 20 studies reported symptom improvement in 77% of patients after radical surgery. Twenty-three per cent of the patients did not improve. Morbidity and mortality were high (26.5 and 1.3%, respectively) [58].

Figure 6 illustrates treatment algorithm for IC/BPS based on the AUA 2022 guidelines [1].

10. Cost of managing IC/BPS

The actual economic burden of IC/BPS on the healthcare system is hard to estimate due to the lack of accurate prevalence. Like other chronic diseases, there are direct and indirect costs. The direct costs include hospital visits, medications, clinical procedures, follow-up, and hospital admission. The average annual cost of managing IC/BPS is higher than the average yearly cost for asthma, depression, diabetes mellitus and hypertension. A study from the United States reported an annual direct cost of $3631 per patient [59].

IC/BPS affects individuals during the most productive period of life. Time away from work and loss of productivity are critical indirect costs that are difficult to calculate but considerable.

The average management cost is higher in women than in men. The extent of indirect costs is proportional to the severity of IC/BPS. The mean annual costs from lost

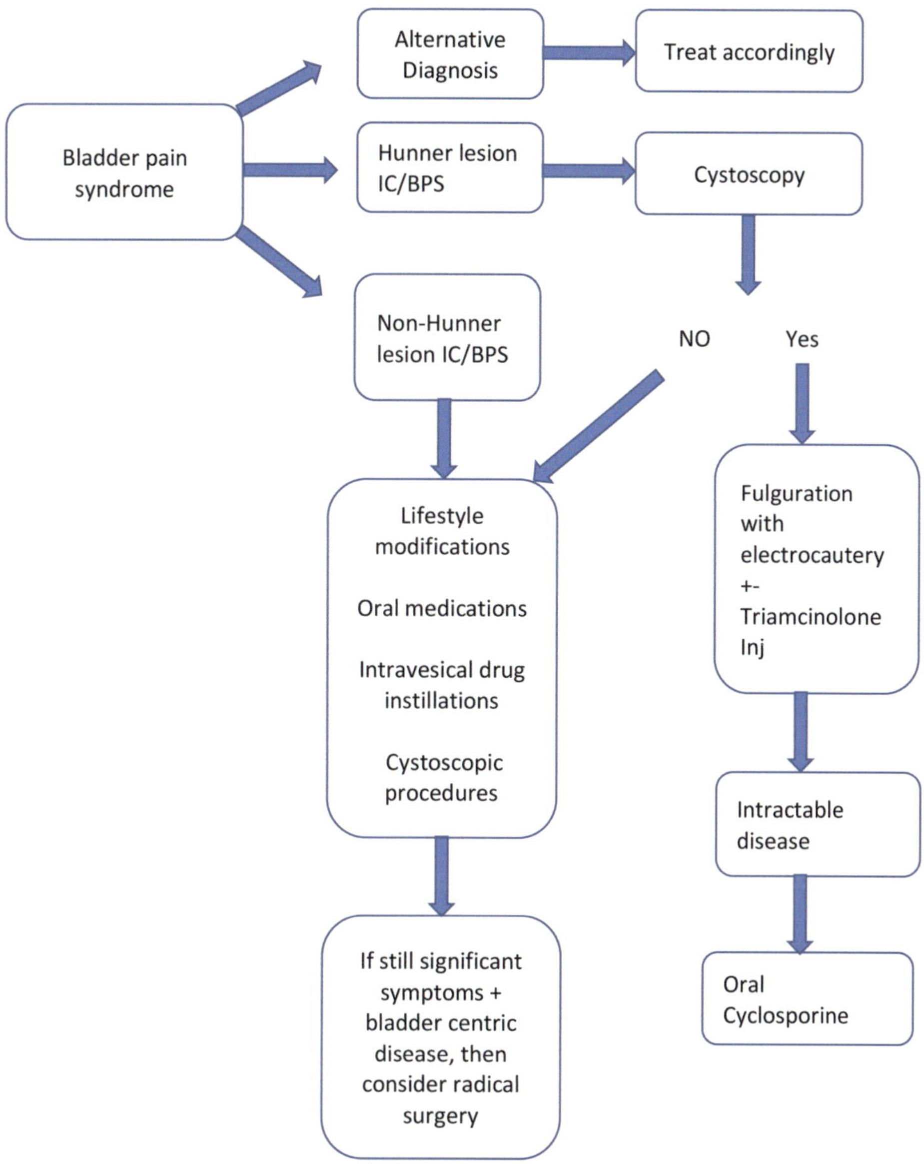

Figure 6.
Algorithm for managing IC/BPS.

wages in the United States were $4216 per patient. Psychological costs, e.g., emotional distress, social isolation, depression, low QoL, and educational and career unpursued activities, are even more difficult to calculate.

11. Drug development and future perspective

The quest for effective therapeutics is ongoing; however, it is slow due to a poor understanding of the IC/BPS pathophysiology. Cannabinoids have anti-inflammatory and analgesic properties and have a role in chronic pain syndromes. The use of cannabinoids in mice cystitis models demonstrated a reduction in pain. Case reports in humans using cannabinoids showed encouraging data.

Tanezumab is a nerve growth factor blocker. It has shown promising results in a small human trial but was associated with toxicity.

Phosphodiesterase-5 inhibitor is a mast cell stabilizer and smooth muscle relaxant. Sildenafil showed improvement in symptoms and urodynamic studies at 3 months.

Roslptor is an inositol-5-phosphatase 1 (SHIP1) activator which modulates the immune system via phosphoinositide signaling. Patients with moderate to severe IC/BPS experienced an improvement in pain and urinary frequency in phase II trials. Unfortunately, favorable effects were lacking in phase III trials.

Hyperbaric oxygen therapy is used in the management of radiation cystitis. It also showed promising results in IC/BPS.

In preclinical work, extracorporeal shock wave therapy (ESWT) improved pain and inflammation. A small, randomized trial of ESWT in IC/BPS showed improvement in the O'Leary-Sant symptoms index and VAS pain score.

Enhanced drug delivery systems deliver the therapeutics to the target area. Using reverse thermal gelation hydrogel has made it possible to use BTX-A without anesthesia. The drug is instilled into the bladder in liquid form. It solidifies in the bladder and releases BTX-A slowly.

Lidocaine releasing intravesical system releases lidocaine over 2 weeks. A pilot study in IC/BPS population reported encouraging results.

Liposomes are biocompatible drug carriers composed of sphingomyelin and phospholipids. Sphingomyelins are part of the cell membrane. A cohort study using intravesical empty liposomes reported improved pain and overall symptoms with no side effects. Liposomes as BTX-A carrier as an alternative to injection therapy was not advantageous.

The promising results of some of these novel experimental therapeutics and drug delivery technologies warrant examination in larger RCTs.

Future research should consider subgroup analysis as a priori or post hoc analysis to assess treatment responses. A urinary or blood biomarker that could diagnose and monitor the treatment effect will be paramount. A prospective registry of IC/BPS patients will provide an excellent platform for understanding the natural history of the disease, risk factors, and the effect of treatments.

12. Conclusions

IC/BPS is a complex chronic condition. The affected patients have a poor quality of life. No test is available to diagnose IC/BPS. It is, therefore, a diagnosis of exclusion. An exception is IC/BPS with Hunner lesion, where cystoscopy is diagnostic. The diagnosis is delayed due to the diagnostic approach. Sometimes it may co-exist with other chronic pain syndromes, which masks the diagnosis. Our understanding of IC/BPS has increased in the last couple of decades. It is now perceived as a chronic pain syndrome.

The treatment paradigm has shifted from bladder-centric therapies to ameliorating symptoms and enhancing the quality of life. Research shows that some therapies are more effective in specific phenotypes. Treatment effects are variable therefore, should be tailored according to the individual patient's needs and resposnse. Complex IC/BPS cases may require a multidisciplinary team approach. There is an unmet medical need for new biomarkers and novel therapeutics.

Acknowledgements

I am thankful to my parents, wife, and children, who supported me during the completion of this chapter. I am also grateful to my supervisor Ida Ryland, who encouraged me to continue my academic work despite the busy clinical work.

No funding was received for this work.

Conflict of interest

The authors declare no conflict of interest.

Notes/thanks/other declarations

I would like to thank one of my IC/BPS patients. She consistently and accurately updated me about her symptoms which assisted me in reaching the diagnosis. Her case was a source of inspiration for researching IC/BPS and writing this chapter.

Appendices and nomenclature

AUA	American Urology Association
BTX-A	botulinum toxin A
CS	chondroitin sulfate
DMSO	dimethyl sulfoxide
ESWT	extracorporeal shock wave therapy
FDA	food and drug administration
FM	fibromyalgia
GAGs	glycosaminoglycans
GUPI	genitourinary pain index
HA	hyaluronic acid
IC/BPS	interstitial cystitis/ Bladder pain syndrome
MAPP	multidisciplinary approach to pelvic pain
MRI	magnetic resonance imaging
NSAIDs	non-steroidal anti-inflammatory drugs
PPS	pentosan polysulphate sodium
PST	potassium sensitivity test
PTNS	percutaneous tibial nerve stimulation
QoL	quality of life
RCT	randomized controlled trial
SNM	sacral neuromodulation
TENS	transcutaneous electrical nerve stimulation
UTI	urinary tract infection
VAS	visual analogue scale
WICI	The University of Wisconsin interstitial cystitis inventory

Author details

Asad Ullah[1*] and Muhammad Jamil[2]

1 University of Liverpool, Liverpool, UK

2 Retired General Practitioner, Peshawar, Pakistan

*Address all correspondence to: drasadullah99@hotmail.com

References

[1] Clemens JQ, Erickson DR, Varela NP, Lai HH. Diagnosis and treatment of interstitial cystitis/bladder pain syndrome. Journal of Urology. 2022;**208**(1):34-42

[2] Payne CK, Joyce GF, Wise M, Clemens JQ. Interstitial cystitis and painful bladder syndrome. The Journal of Urology. 2007;**177**(6):2042-2049

[3] Clemens JQ, Meenan RT, Rosetti MC, Gao SY, Calhoun EA. Prevalence and incidence of interstitial cystitis in a managed care population. The Journal of Urology. 2005;**173**(1):98-102 discussion

[4] Bade JJ, Rijcken B, Mensink HJ. Interstitial cystitis in the Netherlands: Prevalence, diagnostic criteria and therapeutic preferences. The Journal of Urology. 1995;**154**(6):2035-2037 discussion 7-8

[5] Warren JW, Keay SK, Meyers D, Xu J. Concordance of interstitial cystitis in monozygotic and dizygotic twin pairs. Urology. 2001;**57**(6 Suppl 1):22-25

[6] Kairys AE, Schmidt-Wilcke T, Puiu T, Ichesco E, Labus JS, Martucci K, et al. Increased brain gray matter in the primary somatosensory cortex is associated with increased pain and mood disturbance in patients with interstitial cystitis/painful bladder syndrome. The Journal of Urology. 2015;**193**(1):131-137

[7] Misra S, Chetwood A, Coker C, Thomas P. Ketamine cystitis: Practical considerations in management. Scandinavian Journal of Urology. 2014;**48**(5):482-488

[8] Bogart LM, Berry SH, Clemens JQ. Symptoms of interstitial cystitis, painful bladder syndrome and similar diseases in women: A systematic review. The Journal of Urology. 2007;**177**(2):450-456

[9] Propert KJ, Schaeffer AJ, Brensinger CM, Kusek JW, Nyberg LM, Landis JR. A prospective study of interstitial cystitis: Results of longitudinal followup of the interstitial cystitis Data Base cohort. The interstitial cystitis Data Base study group. The Journal of Urology. 2000;**163**(5):1434-1439

[10] Link CL, Pulliam SJ, Hanno PM, Hall SA, Eggers PW, Kusek JW, et al. Prevalence and psychosocial correlates of symptoms suggestive of painful bladder syndrome: Results from the Boston area community health survey. The Journal of Urology. 2008;**180**(2):599-606

[11] Driscoll A, Teichman JMH. How do patients with interstitial cystitis present? Journal of Urology. 2001;**166**(6):2118-2120

[12] Akiyama Y, Luo Y, Hanno PM, Maeda D, Homma Y. Interstitial cystitis/bladder pain syndrome: The evolving landscape, animal models and future perspectives. International Journal of Urology. 2020;**27**(6):491-503

[13] Lai HH, Newcomb C, Harte S, Appleby D, Ackerman AL, Anger JT, et al. Comparison of deep phenotyping features of UCPPS with and without Hunner lesion: A MAPP-II research network study. Neurourology and Urodynamics. 2021;**40**(3):810-818

[14] Tomaszewski JE, Landis JR, Russack V, Williams TM, Wang LP, Hardy C, et al. Biopsy features are associated with primary symptoms in interstitial cystitis: Results from

the interstitial cystitis database study. Urology. 2001;**57**(6 Suppl 1):67-81

[15] Hanno P. Is the potassium sensitivity test a valid and useful test for the diagnosis of interstitial cystitis? Against. International Urogynecology Journal and Pelvic Floor Dysfunction. 2005;**16**(6):428-429

[16] O'Leary MP, Sant GR, Fowler FJ Jr, Whitmore KE, Spolarich-Kroll J. The interstitial cystitis symptom index and problem index. Urology. 1997;**49**(5A Suppl):58-63

[17] Goin JE, Olaleye D, Peters KM, Steinert B, Habicht K, Wynant G. Psychometric analysis of the University of Wisconsin Interstitial Cystitis Scale: Implications for use in randomized clinical trials. The Journal of Urology. 1998;**159**(3):1085-1090

[18] Ware JE Jr. SF-36 health survey update. Spine (Phila Pa 1976). 2000;**25**(24):3130-3139

[19] Parsons CL, Dell J, Stanford EJ, Bullen M, Kahn BS, Waxell T, et al. Increased prevalence of interstitial cystitis: Previously unrecognized urologic and gynecologic cases identified using a new symptom questionnaire and intravesical potassium sensitivity. Urology. 2002;**60**(4):573-578

[20] Nickel JC, Shoskes D, Irvine-Bird K. Clinical phenotyping of women with interstitial cystitis/painful bladder syndrome: A key to classification and potentially improved management. The Journal of Urology. 2009;**182**(1):155-160

[21] Bogart LM, Suttorp MJ, Elliott MN, Clemens JQ, Berry SH. Validation of a quality-of-life scale for women with bladder pain syndrome/interstitial cystitis. Quality of Life Research. 2012;**21**(9):1665-1670

[22] Hebbar S, Pandey H, Chawla A. Understanding King's health questionnaire (KHQ) in assessment of female urinary incontinence. International Journal of Research in Medical Sciences. 2015;**3**(3):531-538

[23] Walker SJ, Zambon J, Andersson KE, Langefeld CD, Matthews CA, Badlani G, et al. Bladder capacity is a biomarker for a bladder centric versus systemic manifestation in interstitial cystitis/ bladder pain syndrome. The Journal of Urology. 2017;**198**(2):369-375

[24] De Gucht V, Heiser W. Alexithymia and somatisation: Quantitative review of the literature. Journal of Psychosomatic Research. 2003;**54**(5):425-434

[25] Friedlander JI, Shorter B, Moldwin RM. Diet and its role in interstitial cystitis/bladder pain syndrome (IC/BPS) and comorbid conditions. BJU International. 2012;**109**(11):1584-1591

[26] Link R. How to follow the interstitial cystitis diet Healthline. 2022 [updated 23-05-2022]. Available from: https://www.healthline.com/nutrition/interstitial-cystitis-diet

[27] Bassaly R, Tidwell N, Bertolino S, Hoyte L, Downes K, Hart S. Myofascial pain and pelvic floor dysfunction in patients with interstitial cystitis. International Urogynecology Journal. 2011;**22**(4):413-418

[28] FitzGerald MP, Payne CK, Lukacz ES, Yang CC, Peters KM, Chai TC, et al. Randomized multicenter clinical trial of myofascial physical therapy in women with interstitial cystitis/painful bladder syndrome and pelvic floor tenderness. The Journal of Urology. 2012;**187**(6):2113-2118

[29] van Ophoven A, Pokupic S, Heinecke A, Hertle L. A prospective,

randomized, placebo controlled, double-blind study of amitriptyline for the treatment of interstitial cystitis. The Journal of Urology. 2004;**172**(2):533-536

[30] Foster HE Jr, Hanno PM, Nickel JC, Payne CK, Mayer RD, Burks DA, et al. Effect of amitriptyline on symptoms in treatment naïve patients with interstitial cystitis/painful bladder syndrome. The Journal of Urology. 2010;**183**(5):1853-1858

[31] Hwang P, Auclair B, Beechinor D, Diment M, Einarson TR. Efficacy of pentosan polysulfate in the treatment of interstitial cystitis: A meta-analysis. Urology. 1997;**50**(1):39-43

[32] Sairanen J, Tammela TL, Leppilahti M, Multanen M, Paananen I, Lehtoranta K, et al. Cyclosporine a and pentosan polysulfate sodium for the treatment of interstitial cystitis: A randomized comparative study. The Journal of Urology. 2005;**174**(6):2235-2238

[33] Nickel JC, Herschorn S, Whitmore KE, Forrest JB, Hu P, Friedman AJ, et al. Pentosan polysulfate sodium for treatment of interstitial cystitis/bladder pain syndrome: Insights from a randomized, double-blind, placebo controlled study. The Journal of Urology. 2015;**193**(3):857-862

[34] van Ophoven A, Vonde K, Koch W, Auerbach G, Maag KP. Efficacy of pentosan polysulfate for the treatment of interstitial cystitis/bladder pain syndrome: Results of a systematic review of randomized controlled trials. Current Medical Research and Opinion. 2019;**35**(9):1495-1503

[35] van Ophoven A, Heinecke A, Hertle L. Safety and efficacy of concurrent application of oral pentosan polysulfate and subcutaneous low-dose heparin for patients with interstitial cystitis. Urology. 2005;**66**(4):707-711

[36] Sant GR, Propert KJ, Hanno PM, Burks D, Culkin D, Diokno AC, et al. A pilot clinical trial of oral pentosan polysulfate and oral hydroxyzine in patients with interstitial cystitis. The Journal of Urology. 2003;**170**(3):810-815

[37] Thilagarajah R, Witherow RO, Walker MM. Oral cimetidine gives effective symptom relief in painful bladder disease: A prospective, randomized, double-blind placebo-controlled trial. BJU International. 2001;**87**(3):207-212

[38] Perez-Marrero R, Emerson LE, Feltis JT. A controlled study of dimethyl sulfoxide in interstitial cystitis. The Journal of Urology. 1988;**140**(1):36-39

[39] Lim YN, Dwyer P, Murray C, Karmakar D, Rosamilia A, Thomas E. Long-term outcomes of intravesical dimethyl sulfoxide/heparin/hydrocortisone therapy for interstitial cystitis/bladder pain syndrome. International Urogynecology Journal. 2017;**28**(7):1085-1089

[40] Tutolo M, Ammirati E, Castagna G, Klockaerts K, Plancke H, Ost D, et al. A prospective randomized controlled multicentre trial comparing intravesical DMSO and chondroïtin sulphate 2% for painful bladder syndrome/interstitial cystitis. International Braz J Urol. 2017;**43**(1):134-141

[41] Nomiya A, Naruse T, Niimi A, Nishimatsu H, Kume H, Igawa Y, et al. On- and post-treatment symptom relief by repeated instillations of heparin and alkalized lidocaine in interstitial cystitis. International Journal of Urology. 2013;**20**(11):1118-1122

[42] Parsons CL, Zupkas P, Proctor J, Koziol J, Franklin A, Giesing D, et al.

Alkalinized lidocaine and heparin provide immediate relief of pain and urgency in patients with interstitial cystitis. The Journal of Sexual Medicine. 2012;**9**(1):207-212

[43] Riedl CR, Engelhardt PF, Daha KL, Morakis N, Pflüger H. Hyaluronan treatment of interstitial cystitis/painful bladder syndrome. International Urogynecology Journal and Pelvic Floor Dysfunction. 2008;**19**(5):717-721

[44] Gülpınar Ö, Esen B, Kayış A, Gökçe M, Süer E. Clinical comparison of intravesical hyaluronic acid and chondroitin sulfate therapies in the treatment of bladder pain syndrome/ interstitial cystitis. Neurourology and Urodynamics. 2018;**37**(1):257-262

[45] Pyo JS, Cho WJ. Systematic review and meta-analysis of Intravesical hyaluronic acid and hyaluronic acid/ chondroitin Sulfate instillation for interstitial cystitis/painful bladder syndrome. Cellular Physiology and Biochemistry. 2016;**39**(4):1618-1625

[46] Barua JM, Arance I, Angulo JC, Riedl CR. A systematic review and meta-analysis on the efficacy of intravesical therapy for bladder pain syndrome/interstitial cystitis. International Urogynecology Journal. 2016;**27**(8):1137-1147

[47] Nickel JC, Moldwin R, Lee S, Davis EL, Henry RA, Wyllie MG. Intravesical alkalinized lidocaine (PSD597) offers sustained relief from symptoms of interstitial cystitis and painful bladder syndrome. BJU International. 2009;**103**(7):910-918

[48] Dunn M, Ramsden PD, Roberts JB, Smith JC, Smith PJ. Interstitial cystitis, treated by prolonged bladder distension. British Journal of Urology. 1977;**49**(7):641-645

[49] Peeker R, Aldenborg F, Fall M. Complete transurethral resection of ulcers in classic interstitial cystitis. International Urogynecology Journal and Pelvic Floor Dysfunction. 2000;**11**(5):290-295

[50] Cox M, Klutke JJ, Klutke CG. Assessment of patient outcomes following submucosal injection of triamcinolone for treatment of Hunner's ulcer subtype interstitial cystitis. The Canadian Journal of Urology. 2009;**16**(2):4536-4540

[51] Lai HH, Pickersgill NA, Vetter JM. Hunner lesion phenotype in interstitial cystitis/bladder pain syndrome: A systematic review and meta-analysis. The Journal of Urology. 2020;**204**(3):518-523

[52] Rofeim O, Hom D, Freid RM, Moldwin RM. Use of the neodymium: YAG laser for interstitial cystitis: A prospective study. The Journal of Urology. 2001;**166**(1):134-136

[53] Kuo HC, Chancellor MB. Comparison of intravesical botulinum toxin type a injections plus hydrodistention with hydrodistention alone for the treatment of refractory interstitial cystitis/painful bladder syndrome. BJU International. 2009;**104**(5):657-661

[54] Forsell T, Ruutu M, Isoniemi H, Ahonen J, Alfthan O. Cyclosporine in severe interstitial cystitis. The Journal of Urology. 1996;**155**(5):1591-1593

[55] Sairanen J, Forsell T, Ruutu M. Long-term outcome of patients with interstitial cystitis treated with low dose cyclosporine a. The Journal of Urology. 2004;**171**(6 Pt 1):2138-2141

[56] Forrest JB, Payne CK, Erickson DR. Cyclosporine a for refractory interstitial

cystitis/bladder pain syndrome: Experience of 3 tertiary centers. The Journal of Urology. 2012;**188**(4):1186-1191

[57] Peters KM, Feber KM, Bennett RC. A prospective, single-blind, randomized crossover trial of sacral vs pudendal nerve stimulation for interstitial cystitis. BJU International. 2007;**100**(4):835-839

[58] Osman NI, Bratt DG, Downey AP, Esperto F, Inman RD, Chapple CR. A systematic review of surgical interventions for the treatment of bladder pain syndrome/interstitial cystitis. European Urology Focus. 2021;7(4):877-885

[59] Clemens JQ, Markossian T, Calhoun EA. Comparison of economic impact of chronic prostatitis/chronic pelvic pain syndrome and interstitial cystitis/painful bladder syndrome. Urology. 2009;**73**(4):743-746

Chapter 5

Radiation Cystitis

Carlos Arturo Levi D'Ancona and André Canettieri Rubez

Abstract

The bladder is incidentally exposed during radiation therapy for cancer involving pelvic structures. Radiation exposure induces urothelium damage and perivascular fibrosis, as well as traumatizes the detrusor smooth muscle, resulting in a decrease in bladder compliance and capacity. The acute and subacute phases of radiation cystitis (RC) occur during or within 3–6 months after therapy. On the other hand, late RC can develop from 6 months to years after radiation treatment. Clinical symptoms may include storage and voiding symptoms, pelvic pain and hematuria. The diagnosis is focused on the exclusion of other causes. The oral therapies include analgesics, anticholinergics, alpha-blockers and 5-reductase inhibitors. Intravesical instillation (e.g., prostaglandin, formalin, hyaluronic acid) have been used for the treatment of late RC. The management of hemorrhagic cystitis is tailored according to the severity of the symptoms, involving conservative measures, hyperbaric oxygen, fulguration, selective embolization, urinary diversion or cystectomy.

Keywords: radiation therapy, lower urinary tract symptoms, cystitis hemorrhagic, radiation cystitis, grade of cystitis

1. Introduction

Radiation is the energy emitted by a source, which is transmitted through a medium and absorbed by another body. For example, high-energy gamma particles can be used for cancer treatment. This therapeutic modality aims to reach high doses of radiation to the target organs, eradicate the tumor and respect the function of the other organs, while preserving the normal tolerance of the surrounding tissues. The treatment of pelvic organ cancers, such as rectal cancer, prostate cancer, uterine cervix cancer or bladder cancer, presents external pelvic radiotherapy as an important therapeutic option [1–3].

Advances in radiation techniques, such as high-energy linear accelerators, intensity-modulated radiotherapy, stereotactic radiotherapy and image-guided brachytherapy, have enabled the administration of increasingly effective doses to the tumor, with an improvement in treatment tolerance, while sparing surrounding tissues. Improved understanding of tissue response to radiation and radiobiological principles has enabled the improvement of fractionation schemes and optimization of the therapeutic ratio between tumor cure and normal tissue damage [1, 2, 4].

Despite the advances, tissue injury still occurs in nontarget organs. The urinary bladder is a critical organ that can be sensitive to low doses of radiation and can be intentionally irradiated in patients with bladder cancer or incidentally in patients with cancer involving other pelvic structures, responsible for acute and/or late adverse events. Bladder injuries and symptoms after irradiation of the pelvic organs define radiation cystitis (RC), and its severity is related to the total dose released, the volume of radiation exposure, the administration scheme and fractionation. Due to the impact on patients' quality of life and the increase in cancer patient survival, a better understanding of the mechanisms of radiation-induced cystitis is essential [2, 4, 5].

Complications associated with radiotherapy account for up to 5–10% of emergency urology admissions. Urinary bladder response to radiation treatment can be classified into acute or subacute reactions occurring within 3–6 months of radiation treatment and late reactions occurring after 6 months to years. Lower urinary tract symptoms are present in these patients. About 5–10% of patients will develop chronic symptoms which remain mild and easily controlled. However, symptoms may persist in a small group of patients and may become debilitating and refractory to conservative treatment [1, 3, 5, 6].

2. Pathophysiology

Radio sensitivity varies in different tissues, largely depending on their proliferative rate [1–5]. The normal epithelium of the bladder is sensitive to radiation and the pathological mechanisms include inflammatory effects of ionizing radiation that damage the urothelium, the detrusor muscle and the vasculature [6]. The radiolysis of water results in the production of activated oxygen free radicals (hydroxyl and superoxide radicals). Cell membrane damage and cell death occur due to lipid peroxidation caused by these highly reactive radicals [1, 7].

Another effect is the genetic damage caused by the absorption of energy by the DNA directly, as well as indirectly by the reaction of the DNA with oxygen radicals. As a consequence, replication defects, mutations and delayed cell death can occur. As a last resort, DNA damage caused by radiation can lead to secondary malignancies [1, 5, 8].

Early symptoms are thought to be caused by injury of the glycosaminoglycan (GAG) layer and the uroepithelium. In general, intermediate and basal urothelial cells show nuclear irregularities and cellular edema, showing signs of damage within the first 3 months after exposure to radiation. Around 6–12 months, an increase in the proliferative activity of the urothelium is observed. The tight junctions and normal proteoglycan layer are disrupted as a result of urothelial radiation injury, which disrupts the barrier between urine and bladder tissue, allowing hypertonic urine and isotonic tissue to come into contact with each other, which results in the appearance of irritative lower urinary tract symptoms that are commonly found early [1, 2, 6].

From 6 months onwards, an increase in vascular endothelial cell proliferation is usually observed, in addition to perivascular fibrosis and vascular thrombosis, potentially resulting in focal ischemia due to vascular occlusion. The smooth muscle of the urinary bladder is also sensitive to radiation. Edema occurs early, usually followed by cell destruction. Vascular ischemia, edema and cell destruction cause the replacement of bladder smooth muscle fibers by fibroblasts, leading to increased collagen deposition (**Figures 1–4**). The result is decreased bladder compliance and functional changes in bladder capacity [5, 6, 8].

Urothelial regeneration and capacity is impaired and results in tissue degradation. Therefore, once the irradiated tissue is injured, effective healing does not occur, making the bladder vulnerable to trauma and infection [3, 4, 7].

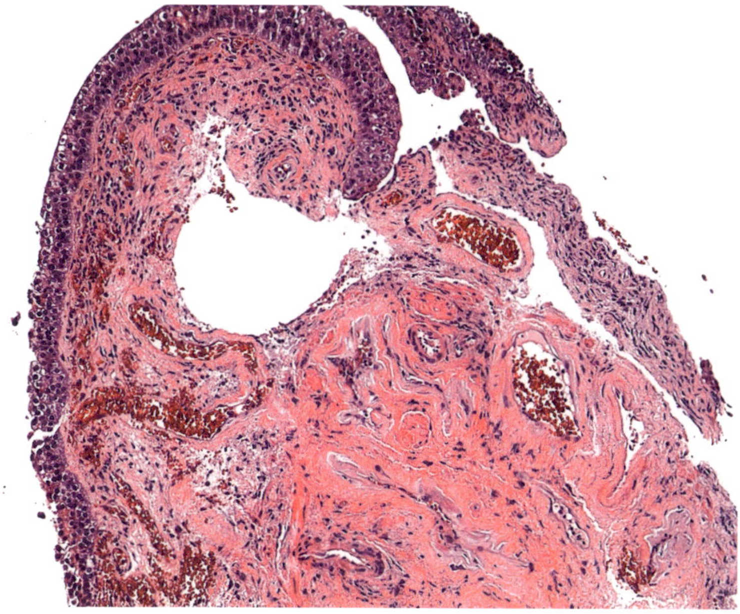

Figure 1.
Perivascular as well as diffuse fibrosis of the vesical mucosa. (Image courtesy of Professor Athanase Billis MD., PhD.).

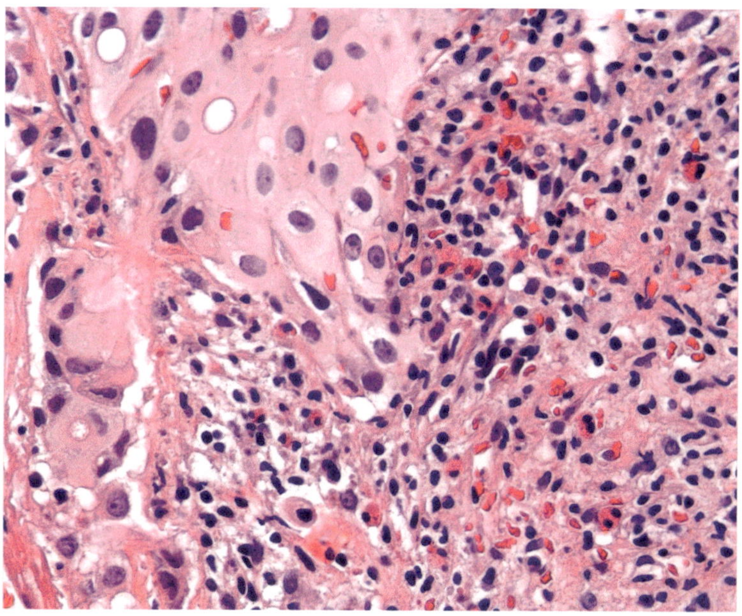

Figure 2.
Dense inflammatory infiltrate with the presence of numerous eosinophils. (Image courtesy of Professor Athanase Billis MD., PhD.).

Vascular endothelial cells are believed to be the main target cell for bladder damage after radiation, particularly in late complications, leading to a range of symptoms including increased urinary frequency, urgency, pelvic pain and hematuria. Changes in

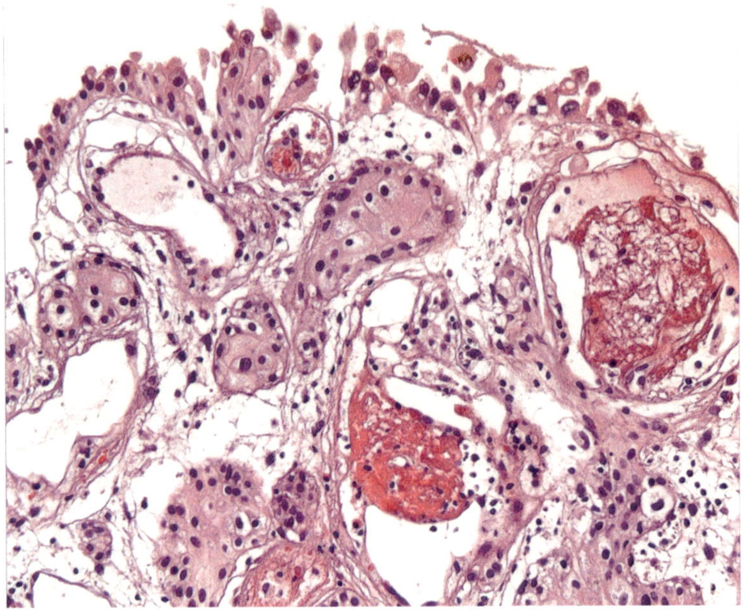

Figure 3.
Vascular thrombosis secondary to radiation lesion of the endothelial cells. (Image courtesy of Professor Athanase Billis MD., PhD.).

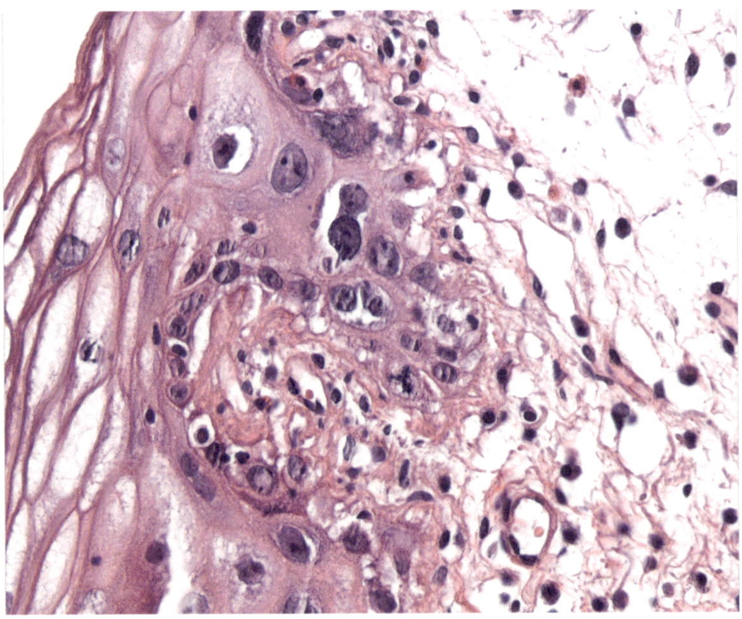

Figure 4.
Intense nuclear atypia in the urothelium and edema in the vesical mucosa. (Image courtesy of Professor Athanase Billis MD., PhD.).

endothelial cells are observed months to years after radiotherapy. Injury to the epithelial cell layer does not appear to play a major role in the development of late effects [1, 5, 6, 8, 9]. Endoscopic view of late radiation damage of vesical mucosa (**Figures 5** and **6**).

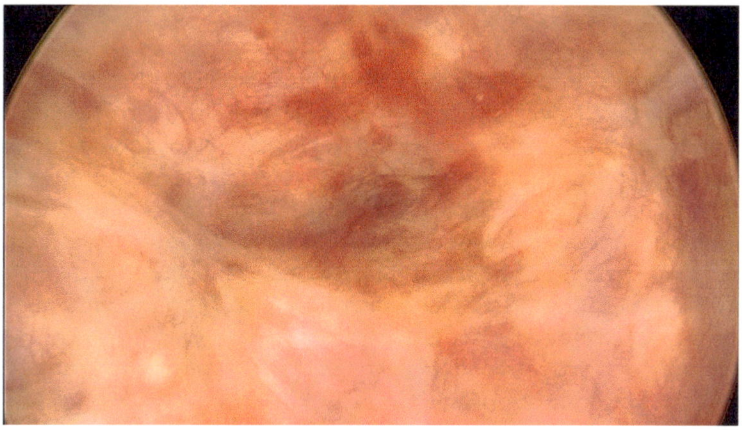

Figure 5.
Cystoscopic findings: erythema, edema, bleeding ulcers and fibrosis (with reduced bladder capacity).

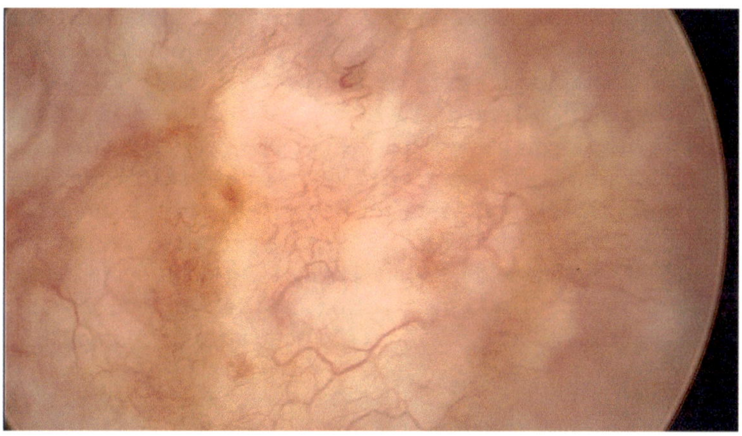

Figure 6.
Cystoscopic findings: atrophic mucosa with telangiectatic blood vessels.

3. Clinical presentation

3.1 Acute radiation cystitis

The definition of acute RC is any clinical manifestation that is provoked during or up to 3 months after the end of radiotherapy. Its side effects are experienced by almost half of the patients after pelvic irradiation in full curative doses. Clinical symptoms include storage and voiding symptoms, such as increased urinary frequency, nocturia, urinary urgency, dysuria, cystalgia with bladder spasms, and (rarely) hematuria. Acute symptoms are mainly caused by injury to the bladder mucosa, which causes a lesion in the urothelial, involving an inflammatory response and tissue edema, leaving the bladder susceptible to trauma and infection. In most cases, this condition is self-limiting and the prognosis is favorable, usually disappearing spontaneously within 6 weeks after the end of radiotherapy [2, 3, 10, 11].

3.2 Chronic radiation cystitis

Late RC can develop after as little as 3 months and possibly up to several years after the end of radiotherapy. Appears on average over the next 2–3 years. Toxicities that occur between 3 and 6 months are sometimes defined as "early delay." Late symptomatology after radiotherapy for cancers in the pelvic region has an incidence of 5–10% despite improved techniques and is more common in patients with bladder cancer treated with radiation. The clinical presentation can be variable, including lower urinary tract symptoms, but the most characteristic clinical feature is recurrent hematuria, with variable severity, which can be fatal in more severe cases [8, 10, 12–14]. The injury caused is progressive, and the compromised tissue is susceptible to secondary urinary tract infection and minor trauma, which due to poor healing, can lead to ulcers and eventual perforation of the bladder in addition to the formation of fistulas. During the investigation, these lesions may be aggravated by inappropriate bladder biopsies, and should therefore be avoided in previously irradiated areas. Pre-existing medical conditions such as diabetes, hypertension, previous unrelated abdominal surgery, and patients receiving concomitant chemotherapy are important risk factors. The most important factors are those related to radiation treatment, including the volume of tissue treated, total bladder dose and fractionation, route of delivery (external beam and/or brachytherapy), concomitant treatments and the radiosensitivity of the affected bladder tissue. After high-dose exposures (such as after brachytherapy treatment), some areas of the bladder may be at greater risk of injury, such as the bladder neck. Therefore, it is important to identify patients with risk factors for developing a severe form [1, 5, 13, 14]. Fibrosis of the bladder wall with reduced urinary capacity can occur up to 10 years after radiotherapy. These changes predispose to the appearance of neovascularization in the form of telangiectasias and bladder bleeding, in addition to lower urinary tract symptoms that are partially related to interstitial and smooth muscle fibrosis and reduced bladder capacity. Hematuria is the main presenting symptom and can range from mild hematuria to life-threatening hemorrhage. Hematuria with clot formation can lead to urinary retention [5, 10, 12].

4. Diagnosis

Diagnosis of RC is based primarily on excluding other causes of hematuria and the patient's symptoms, as the clinical features are nonspecific and may also be caused by bladder infection or malignancy. An initial evaluation involves a complete patient history and physical examination. Diagnostic evaluation for hematuria includes urinalysis, urine culture and antibiogram to exclude infection. Urine cytology is valuable for detecting high-grade malignancy, but UTI must be interpreted with caution, as changes from prior radiotherapy can be a confounding factor. Imaging evaluation by ultrasonography, excretory urography, or computed tomography (CT) can exclude an upper tract lesion as the cause of hematuria, and magnetic resonance imaging (MRI) should be considered in the presence of a previous pelvic malignancy. The most important exam in this phase is the evaluation of the lower urinary tract in the form of cystoscopy, which may reveal atrophic mucosa with telangiectatic blood vessels, erythema, edema, bleeding ulcers, fistulas or fibrosis with reduced bladder capacity (**Figures 5** and **6**). At the time of cystoscopy, bladder biopsy may be performed if tumor recurrence is suspected, with special attention to the potential risk of perforation of the irradiated bladder wall. The biopsy should also be interpreted with the knowledge that changes resulting from previous radiotherapy can be confused with malignancy [1, 5, 12, 13, 15].

5. Grading

The EORTC (European Organization for Research and Treatment of Cancer) and RTOG (Radiation Therapy Oncology Group) have developed uniform scales of radiation toxicity in different target organs, which are standardized and include the subjective, objective, managerial and analytical (SOMA) assessment of late effects in normal tissues (LENT). Each organ or tissue that is within the target zone of irradiation and at risk of being injured has its own LENT-SOMA scale based on the original RTOG criteria for radiation morbidity. The LENT-SUM scale is a comprehensive system scale and provides a lot of information, but it is not practical and difficult to implement routinely outside of clinical trials. Alternatively, the severity of hematuria can be graded using RTOG/EORTC9 and NCI CTCAE (National Cancer Institute Common Terminology Criteria for Adverse Events) grading systems, which are likely to be more practical to use and therefore more widely used in clinical practice [16–19].

Radiation complications involving the bladder are graded on a scale devised by the RTOG. The scale is as follows:

- Grade 1—Any slight epithelial atrophy, microscopic hematuria and mild telangiectasia
- Grade 2—Any moderate frequency, generalized telangiectasia, intermittent macroscopic hematuria and intermittent incontinence
- Grade 3—Any severe frequency and urgency, severe telangiectasia, persistent incontinence, reduced bladder capacity (<150 ml) and frequent hematuria
- Grade 4—Any necrosis, fistula and hemorrhagic cystitis, bladder capacity (<100 ml), refractory incontinence requiring catheter or surgical intervention
- Grade 5—Death.

6. Treatment

There are several treatment options for RC. However, the dearth of high-quality evidence in the form of randomized controlled trials hampers the development of treatment algorithms. Management strategies can be divided into systemic treatments, intravesical treatments, ablative, hyperbaric and interventional procedures such as definitive surgeries. The objective of the treatment and the modality chosen depend on the symptoms presented by the patient and the stage of the disease [1, 3, 5, 10].

In acute phase, the standard management is conservative, aiming at symptomatic control with the use of anticholinergic drugs with the aim of decreasing detrusor contractility and symptomatic improvement. Alpha-blockers, 5-reductase inhibitors or phosphodiesterase 5 inhibitors may be prescribed for the relief of voiding symptoms. Interruption of radiotherapy may be considered in case of severe symptoms. However, we must consider that such interruption in the treatment can influence the control of the tumor [2, 3, 10, 11].

General behavioral guidelines are part of the treatment, good hydration is recommended in order to increase diuresis, it can limit discomfort, in addition to preventing urinary obstruction resulting from blood clots. The use of analgesics and anti-inflammatories for a short period of time period of time, can be indicated. Phosphodiesterase type 5 inhibitors include tadalafil, originally prescribed for the treatment of erectile dysfunction, its mechanism of action in improving irrigation of the bladder is still not clearly elucidated, and it should be remembered that concomitant use with nitrates is formally contraindicated [10, 16, 20].

The biggest challenge in the management of a patient with RC is hematuria. There are a variety of treatment options. Initial management is continuous bladder irrigation should be started after a three-way transurethral catheter is inserted which is continued until the urine is clear. In case of severe hematuria includes patient resuscitation, and if the hemorrhagic shock is present, aggressive intravenous fluid replacement is required, and blood transfusion is indicated. In refractory cases of hematuria require alternative treatment options, which will be discussed below [1, 3, 5, 9, 10].

6.1 Systemic therapies

The aim of systemic treatments is to replace or augment the polysaccharide layer of the bladder and reduce vascular fragility. WF10 is an intravenous formulation, a chemically stabilized chlorite-matrix manufactured from the drug substance OXO K993, also known as tetrachlorodecaoxygen, which has been shown to have a positive effect on chronic inflammatory conditions. Its mechanism of action is based on the model of a postirradiated bladder in a state of chronic inflammation. It induces natural immunity and stimulates cellular defense mechanisms through its action on natural killer cells, cytotoxic T lymphocytes and modification of the monocyte-macrophage system. It reduces inflammation quickly so healing can begin. It is a promising therapy, with studies showing a response rate of up to 80%. Veerasarn et al. showed that patients treated with WF10 (n = 37) had a significantly lower rate of recurrence of recurrent hematuria after 12 months (47% vs. 77%; P = 0.01). Side effects include nausea, headache and transient anemia. Until now, the WF10 is not currently licensed for the treatment of RC [21–23].

Sodium pentosan polysulfate is a synthetic sulfated polysaccharide believed to adhere to the surface of the bladder and is used to decrease urothelial permeability by replacing defective GAGs. Sandhu et al. recommended its use as the primary method of management of pelvic radiotherapy-associated hemorrhagic cystitis based on their experience with administering oral pentosan polysulfate sodium 100 mg three times daily to control radiation-induced hemorrhagic cystitis in 60 patients. The dose was gradually reduced to a maintenance dose of 100 mg in 21 patients who had a partial response. At the end of the study, 10 patients had a complete response. One limitation was the "time to effect," as the onset of action was from 1 to 8 weeks. During this period, 15 patients required hospitalization for bladder irrigation [24].

Corticosteroids have not been widely used in the treatment of hemorrhagic RC. However, in the literature, we found reports of remission of hematuria obtained only after treatment with dexamethasone. Furthermore, a beneficial effect of glucocorticoids in the treatment of ifosfamide-induced hemorrhagic cystitis has been demonstrated. Corticosteroids can be beneficial for hemorrhagic cystitis by improving hematologic parameters by promoting erythropoiesis [25, 26].

Tranexamic acid has been used to treat hematuria and can be given in the early stages of conservative management of active bleeding in patients with prior radiotherapy, although evidence of efficacy in this group of patients is lacking.

Tranexamic acid acts by inhibiting fibrinolysis; therefore, it can lead to the formation of large clots with consequent urinary retention. Its use has been associated with an increased risk of thromboembolic events. It can be considered in bleeding; however, complications of clot retention limit its use [27].

6.2 Hyperbaric oxygenation

Hyperbaric oxygen therapy enhances oxygen delivery to tissues by increasing the amount of dissolved oxygen in plasma to induce and restore normal repair of granulocytes and fibroblasts, inducing neoangiogenesis with the restoration of ≤80% of capillary density. The usual course of treatment involves 35–40 sessions of 90–100 minutes each, 5 days a week, breathing 100% oxygen at 2 atmospheres of absolute pressure per session. Success rates range from 76% to 95% for short-term results and 72–83% for long-term results, where success is defined as symptomatic and/or cystoscopic improvement in RC [28–30].

6.3 Intravesical therapies

Response rates with intravesical therapies generally range from 60% to 90%. Formalin and alum instillations are historically evidence-based intravesical therapies for the treatment of hemorrhagic RC. Formalin precipitates cellular proteins within the epithelial layer, and this leads to fixation of friable and telangiectatic microvasculature occlusion. However, contemporary evidence is limited on the use of formalin, and devastating complications, such as patient mortality, have been described. Formalin is only recommended in cases of intractable hemorrhagic cystitis that may require urinary diversion [31]. Aluminum salts, such as potassium or ammonium aluminum sulfate, act by precipitating proteins on the surface of cells. Intravesical instillation of alum is not as effective as formalin; however, it has fewer side effects and may represent an early treatment option if more conservative initial measures are unsuccessful. Hyaluronic acid is an important mucopolysaccharide that can be instilled into the urinary bladder and is part of new intravesical therapies that aim to replace the protective layer of GAG to reduce the exposure of underlying epithelial cells to urine. It has immunomodulatory properties that improve the healing of connective tissue. Epsilon aminocaproic acid can be instilled into the bladder and inhibits fibrinolysis to neutralize urokinase in telangiectatic vessels. Several other agents, including prostaglandins, botulinum toxin, polydeoxyribonucleotides and early placental extract, have also been reported, with limited response rates [6, 10].

Tacrolimus acts as a potent immunosuppressant that improves the barrier function of the skin and mucosa, in addition to inducing local vasoconstriction. It is a calcineurin inhibitor that hinders the production and release of pro-inflammatory cytokines in T cells. Although systemic administration has a high incidence of adverse events, when used specifically locally, minimal adverse events occur. This effect led to studies investigating intravesical instillation of tacrolimus as a possible treatment for radiation hemorrhagic cystitis. The effect of liposomal tacrolimus was also observed in the model of cyclophosphamide-induced hemorrhagic cystitis [32, 33].

6.4 Ablative therapies

Ablation techniques and coagulation with laser therapy or argon-beam therapies are methods that can immediately control bleeding. Although there is a need for general or spinal anesthesia, they are associated with a complete response in 75–97% [3]. The Green Light LASER spares the surrounding tissue as it can ablate blood vessels with selective absorption of green light by intravascular oxyhemoglobin. In contrast, the YAG laser is not selective and has an increased risk of bladder perforation [34]. In the case of argon-beam coagulation, an argon probe is directed approximately 3 mm from the vessel and a monopolar current is directed through it and has a safety mechanism to prevent perforation. The depth of ablation can be changed by adjusting the settings of energy and gas flow. In addition, the current follows the path of least resistance and moves to the adjacent tissue after coagulation has been achieved [35].

6.5 Interventional radiologic

Despite limited evidence of its use in the treatment of hemorrhagic RC, arterial embolization may be a therapeutic possibility. Small series of cases describe its use, with the resolution of hematuria ranging from 90% to 100% and depending on the group of patients [36, 37]. Ischemic complications occur in 10–62.5% of patients and may include skin or bladder necrosis, gluteal paresis, Brown-Sequard syndrome and perineal or buttock pain, depending on the selectivity of embolization [3, 36].

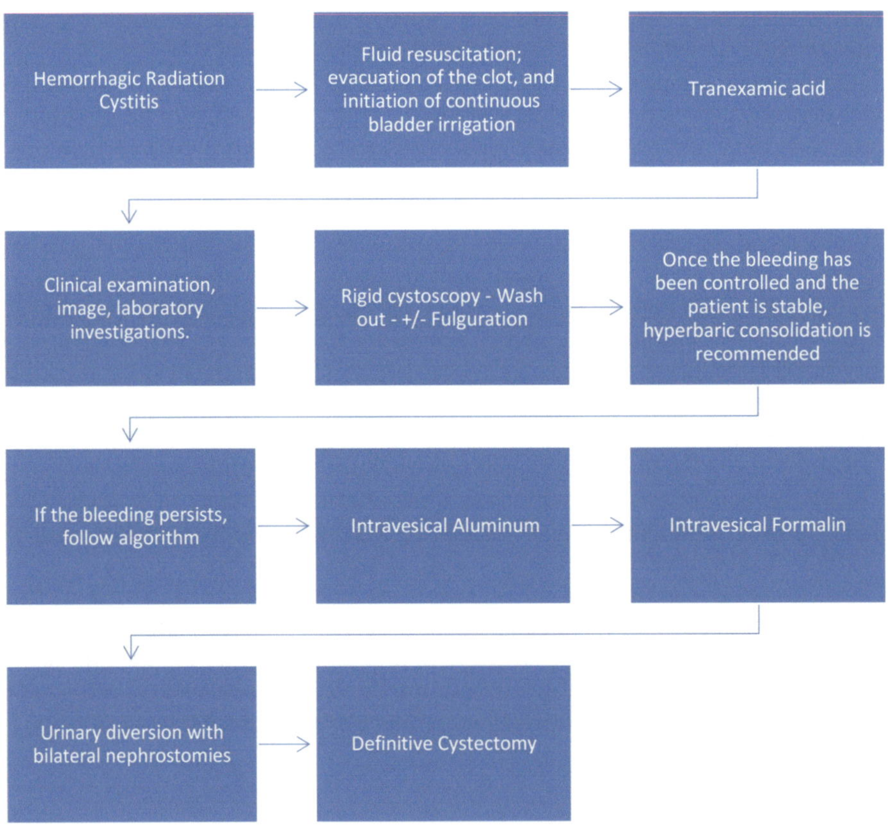

Figure 7.
Algorithm for radiation-induced hemorrhagic cystitis illustrating the recommended practical management.

6.6 Definitive surgical treatment

If all other less invasive treatment methods fail, urinary diversion with or without cystectomy can be performed. However, this approach has high morbidity. A series of 21 patients undergoing cystectomy and urinary diversion for intractable hemorrhagic cystitis showed that 42% of patients developed a Grade III or IV ClavienDindo complication. Furthermore, the 3-month mortality rate was 16% [38].

There are no widely adopted definitive clinical approach algorithms for managing patients with radiation-induced hematuria. The stepwise, evidence-based approach to the treatment of this patient population can be found in **Figure 7**.

As important as management are strategies to reduce the effects on the urinary tract, such as performing radiotherapy sessions with a full bladder (except in cases of bladder cancer in which this is not possible). In addition, there has been increasing interest in the use of stereotactic body radiation therapy (SBRT). The main advantage is that the treatment, based on image-guided approaches with narrow margins, is done in five fractions (750–800 cGy per fraction), with lower doses for adjacent organs at risk. Biochemical control was comparable to standard IMRT, and treatment morbidity was low [2, 4, 39].

7. Conclusion

Currently, high-quality evidence describing the management of RC is scarce. Acute radiation injury to the bladder is usually self-limiting; however, delayed RC, although relatively rare, can lead to severe bleeding and can be difficult to treat. In the absence of robust evidence for any treatment modality, most patients are managed supportively in the first instance and most patients require multimodal treatment. Numerous treatment options have been studied over the last few decades, but many patients still require surgery to stop life-threatening hematuria. Surgery of this nature is often associated with significant morbidity, and any alternative treatment options should be further explored. In the future, large randomized trials that explore emerging management strategies are needed to strengthen evidence-based treatment strategies.

Author details

Carlos Arturo Levi D'Ancona[1*] and André Canettieri Rubez[2]

1 Full Professor of Urology, School of Medical Science, University of Campinas, São Paulo, Brazil

2 Resident of Urology, School of Medical Science, University of Campinas, São Paulo, Brazil

*Address all correspondence to: cdancona@uol.com.br

References

[1] Smit SG, Heyns CF. Management of radiation cystitis. Nature Reviews Urology. 2010;**7**(4):206-214. DOI: 10.1038/nrurol.2010.23. Epub 2010 Mar 9

[2] Marks LB, Carroll PR, Dugan TC, Anscher MS. The response of the urinary bladder, urethra, and ureter to radiation and chemotherapy. International Journal of Radiation Oncology, Biology, Physics. 1995;**31**(5):1257-1280. DOI: 10.1016/0360-3016(94)00431-J

[3] Pascoe C, Duncan C, Lamb BW, Davis NF, Lynch TH, Murphy DG, Lawrentschuk N. Current management of radiation cystitis: a review and practical guide to clinical management. BJU International 2019;**123**(4):585-594. DOI: 10.1111/bju.14516. Epub 2018 Nov 28

[4] Mühlstädt S, Mohammed N, Weigand K, Schumann A, Kawan F, Göllert C, et al. Radiogen bedingte Zystitis: Pathophysiologie und Therapie [Radiation cystitis: pathophysiology and treatment]. Urologe A. 2017;**56**(3):301-305. German. DOI: 10.1007/s00120-017-0319-2

[5] Crew JP, Jephcott CR, Reynard JM. Radiation-induced haemorrhagic cystitis. European Urology. 2001;**40**(2):111-123. DOI: 10.1159/000049760

[6] Browne C, Davis NF, Mac Craith E, Lennon GM, Mulvin DW, Quinlan DM, et al. A narrative review on the pathophysiology and management for radiation cystitis. Adv Urol. 2015;**2015**:346812. DOI: 10.1155/2015/346812 Epub 2015 Dec 22

[7] Del Pizzo JJ, Chew BH, Jacobs SC, Sklar GN. Treatment of radiation induced hemorrhagic cystitis with hyperbaric oxygen: long-term followup. Journal of Urology. 1998;**160** (3 Part 1):731-733

[8] Shah SK, Lui PD, Baldwin DD, Ruckle HC. Urothelial carcinoma after external beam radiation therapy for prostate cancer. Journal of Urology. 2006;**175**(6):2063-2066. DOI: 10.1016/S0022-5347(06)00324-7

[9] Dautruche A, Delouya G. A contemporary review about the management of radiation-induced hemorrhagic cystitis. Current Opinion in Supportive and Palliative Care. 2018 Sep;**12**(3):344-350. DOI: 10.1097/SPC.0000000000000375

[10] Helissey C, Cavallero S, Brossard C, Dusaud M, Chargari C, François S. Chronic inflammation and radiation-induced cystitis: molecular background and therapeutic perspectives. Cell. 2020;**10**(1):21. DOI: 10.3390/cells10010021

[11] Mazeron R, Castelnau-Marchand P, Dumas I, Del Campo ER, Kom LK, Martinetti F, et al. Impact of treatment time and dose escalation on local control in locally advanced cervical cancer treated by chemoradiation and image-guided pulsed-dose rate adaptive brachytherapy. Radiotherapy and Oncology. 2015;**114**:257-263

[12] Levenback C, Eifel PJ, Burke TW, Morris M, Gershenson DM. Hemorrhagic cystitis following radiotherapy for stage Ib cancer of the cervix. Gynecologic Oncology. 1994;**55**:206-210

[13] Sun R, Koubaa I, Limkin EJ, Dumas I, Bentivegna E, Castanon E, et al. Locally advanced cervical cancer with bladder invasion: clinical outcomes and

predictive factors for vesicovaginal fistulae. Oncotarget. 2018;**9**:9299-9310

[14] Manea E, Escande A, Bockel S, Khettab M, Dumas I, Lazarescu I, et al. Risk of late urinary complications following image guided adaptive brachytherapy for locally advanced cervical cancer: refining bladder dose-volume parameters. International Journal of Radiation Oncology, Biology, Physics. 2018;**101**:411-420

[15] Mendenhall WM, Henderson RH, Costa JA, Hoppe BS, Dagan R, Bryant CM, et al. Hemorrhagic radiation cystitis. American Journal of Clinical Oncology. 2015;**38**:331-336

[16] Pavy J-J et al. Late effects toxicity scoring: the SOMA scale. International Journal of Radiation Oncology, Biology, Physics. 1995;**31**:1043-1047

[17] Power DA. Late effects of radiotherapy: how to assess and improve outcomes. The British Journal of Radiology. 2005;**78**:150-152

[18] De vries CR, Freiha FS. Hemorrhagic cystitis: a review. Journal of Urology 1990;**143**:1-9

[19] National Cancer Institute. Cancer Therapy Evaluation Program: Protocol Development [online]. 2009. Available from: http://ctep.cancer.gov/protocolDevelopment/electronic_applications/ctc.htm

[20] Rehailia-Blanchard A, He MY, Rancoule C, Guillaume É, Guy J-B, Vial N, et al. Medical prevention and treatment of radiation-induced urological and nephrological complications. Cancer radiotherapie: journal de la Societe francaise de radiotherapie oncologique. 2019;**23**:151-160

[21] Veerasarn V, Khorprasert C, Lorvidhaya V, et al. Reduced recurrence of late hemorrhagic radiation cystitis by WF10 therapy in cervical cancer patients: a multicenter, randomized, two-arm, open-label trial. Radiotherapy and Oncology. 2004;**73**(2):179-185

[22] Veerasarn V, Boonnuch W, Kakanaporn C. A phase II study to evaluate WF10 in patients with late hemorrhagic radiation cystitis and proctitis. Gynecologic Oncology. 2006;**100**(1):179-184

[23] Srisupundit S, Kraiphibul P, Sangruchi S, Linasmita V, Chingskol K, Veerasarn V. The efficacy of chemicallystabilized chlorite-matrix (TCDO) in the management of late postradiation cystitis. Journal of the Medical Association of Thailand. 1999;**82**:798-802

[24] Sandhu SS, Goldstraw M, Woodhouse CR. The management of haemorrhagic cystitis with sodium pentosan polysulphate. BJU International. 2004;**94**:845-847

[25] Jin JG. High-dose methylprednisolone is effective in treating radiation-induced refractory haemorrhagic cystitis. Internal Medicine Journal. 2014;**44**(6):615-617

[26] Liem X, Saad F, G. Delouya.A practical approach to the management of radiation-induced hemorrhagic cystitis. Drugs. 2015;**75**(13):1471-1482

[27] Reed R, Woolley T. Uses of tranexamic acid. Continuing Education in Anaesthesia Critical Care & Pain. 2015;**15**:32-37

[28] Oliai C, Fisher B, Jani A, et al. Hyperbaric oxygen therapy for radiation-induced cystitis and proctitis. International Journal of

Radiation Oncology, Biology, Physics. 2012;**84**(3):733740

[29] Chong KT, Hampson NB, Corman JM. Early hyperbaric oxygen therapy improves outcome for radiation induced hemorrhagic cystitis. Urology. 2005;**65**(4):649653

[30] Oscarsson N, Arnell P, Lodding P, Ricksten S-E, Seeman-Lodding H. Hyperbaric oxygen treatment in radiationinduced cystitis and proctitis: a prospective cohort study on patient-perceived quality of recovery. International Journal of Radiation Oncology Biology Physics. 2013;**87**(4):670-675

[31] Denton AS, Clarke NW, Maher EJ. Non-surgical interventions for late radiation cystitis in patients who have received radical radiotherapy to the pelvis. Cochrane Database of Systematic Reviews 2002; CD001773

[32] Rajaganapathy BR, Janicki JJ, Levanovich P, Tyagi P, Hafron J, Chancellor MB, et al. Intravesical liposomal tacrolimus protects against radiation cystitis induced by 3-beam targeted bladder radiation. Journal of Urology. 2015;**194**(2):578-584. DOI: 10.1016/j.juro.2015.03.108 Epub 2015 Apr 1

[33] Chuang YC, Tyagi P, Huang HY, Yoshimura N, Wu M, Kaufman J, Chancellor MB. Intravesical immune suppression by liposomal tacrolimus in cyclophosphamide-induced inflammatory cystitis. Neurourology and Urodynamics 2011;**30**(3):421-427. DOI: 10.1002/nau.20981. Epub 2010 Sep 21

[34] Talab SS, McDougal WS, Wu CL, Tabatabaei S. Mucosa-sparing, KTP laser coagulation of submucosal telangiectatic vessels in patients with radiation-induced cystitis: a novel approach. Urology. 2014;**84**:47883

[35] Wines MP, Lynch WD. A new minimally invasive technique for treating radiation cystitis: the argon-beam coagulator. BJU International. 2006;**98**:610-612

[36] Delgal A, Cercueil JP, Koutlidis N, et al. Outcome of transcatheter arterial embolization for bladder and prostate hemorrhage. Journal of Urology. 2010;**183**:1947-1953

[37] Korkmaz M, Sanal B, Aras B, et al. The short- and long-term effectiveness of transcatheter arterial embolization in patients with intractable hematuria. Diagnostic and Interventional Imaging. 2016;**97**:197-201

[38] Linder BJ, Tarrell RF, Boorjian SA. Cystectomy for refractory hemorrhagic cystitis: contemporary etiology, presentation and outcomes. Journal of Urology. 2014;**192**:1687-1692

[39] Kishan AU, Dang A, Katz AJ, et al. Long-term outcomes of stereotactic body radiotherapy for low-risk and intermediate-risk prostate cancer. JAMA Network Open. 2019;**2**(2):e188006. DOI: 10.1001/jamanetworkopen.2018.8006

Chapter 6

Drug-Related Cystitis: An Overview

Seçkin Engin

Abstract

Cystitis is an inflammatory condition of the urinary bladder with infectious or noninfectious aetiologies. Chemical-induced cystitis represents a relatively highly prevalent kind of noninfectious cystitis resulting from therapeutic agents or environmental chemicals. Drug-related cystitis is a type of urotoxicity of drugs, which is a commonly underreported condition leading to impaired quality of patients' life, discontinuation of medication and non-compliance. Drug-related cystitis can occur in several forms ranging from mild urinary symptoms to gross haematuria, which can be challenging for physicians to treat. Chemotherapeutic drugs, ketamine, tiaprofenic acid and several drugs have been reported to be associated with cystitis until now. Cyclophosphamide (CP) is an alkylating agent that leads to haemorrhagic cystitis with widespread awareness due to its high prevalence in patients under treatment intravenously. However, several currently available drugs have been also reported to induce cystitis, which may be usually ignored. Drug-related cystitis can cause emergency admissions and prolonged hospitalisation, leading to increased medical costs. Some cases of drug-related cystitis are clinically managed with established therapeutic interventions and/or prophylaxis, such as CP-induced haemorrhagic cystitis. On the other hand, standard treatment is currently unavailable for most cases. This chapter will provide current knowledge regarding the drug-related cystitis that should be taken into consideration as a potential adverse effect of drugs by physicians.

Keywords: adverse effect, bladder, case reports, cystitis, patient compliance, urotoxicity

1. Introduction

Cystitis is a clinical term that is used to refer to the inflammation of the urinary bladder with various aetiologies related to microbial infection, drugs, environmental chemicals and irradiation [1]. Cystitis may be induced by usage of several drugs, making the patients suffer from urinary symptoms such as dysuria, frequency and urgency in the absence or presence of haematuria [2]. Although the prevalence of drug-related cystitis is quite diverse, alkylating chemotherapeutic agents are the most frequently associated with cystitis [1]. Besides certain drugs with well-described urotoxicity, drug-related cystitis is a commonly underreported condition, resulting in non-compliance, drug discontinuation and prolonged hospitalisation [3]. Chemotherapeutics, ketamine, tiaprofenic acid and several drugs have been reported to cause cystitis until now (**Table 1**). There is currently no standard to diagnose

• Cyclophoshamide • Ifosfamide • Ketamine • Tiaprofenic acid • Penicillins ○ Pencillin G ○ Methicillin ○ Carbenicillin ○ Ticarcillin ○ Piperacillin	• Immune checkpoint inhibitors ○ Ipilimumab ○ Atezolizumab ○ Nivolumab ○ Pembrolizumab ○ Sintilimab • Bacillus Calmette Guerin	• Miscellaneous drugs o Busulfan o Thiotepa o Temozolomide o Dacarbazine o Doxorubicin o Epirubicin o Valrubicin o Ethoglucid o Cisplatin o Mitoxantrone o Docetaxel o Paclitaxel o Cabazitaxel o Gefitinib o Indomethacin	o Diclofenac o Ketoprofen o Naproxen o Piroxicam o Atorvastatin o Empagliflozin o Acetylsalicylic o acid o Dabigatran o Allopurinol o Danazol o Methaqualone o Methenamine mandelate

Table 1.
Drugs have been associated with cystitis.

drug-related cystitis, in which its diagnosis usually relies on cystoscopy and clinical presentation along with the exclusion of other aetiologies such as infection, radiation-induced cystitis and metastasis [1]. There are available approved therapeutic or prophylactic regimens for CP or ifosfamide (IFO)-induced cystitis. However, several cases of drug-related cystitis still lack of standard treatment regimen, leading to a challenge to manage [1, 4]. As a general approach, the discontinuation of suspected drugs and glucocorticoids are used to treat drug-related cystitis [2, 5]. Therefore, clinicians should be aware of drug-related cystitis in patients with urinary discomfort that may be urotoxic side effects of the drugs.

2. Cyclophosphamide and Ifosfamide

Cyclophosphamide (CP) is an alkylating agent that is extensively used for the treatment of lymphomas and solid tumours. Although initially approved for malignancies, CP is now utilised in various autoimmune diseases due to its immunomodulatory effects. CP is a prodrug rapidly metabolised to 4-hydroxycyclophosphamide by hepatic cytochrome P450 (CYP) enzymes in particular CYP2B6 and CYP2C19. 4-hydroxycyclophosphamide coexists with its tautomer, aldophosphamide is cleaved intracellularly to form phosphoramide mustard that is responsible for the cytotoxic effect of CP via cross-linking DNA strands, leading to the inhibition of the proliferation of malignant cells [6, 7].

CP still remains one of the most effective drugs to treat various types of malignancies, however, CP is usually associated with a diverse spectrum of complications including gonadal toxicity, nephrotoxicity, hepatotoxicity, pulmonary toxicity, cardiac toxicity, haematological toxicities, secondary malignancies and urotoxicity, which limits its clinical utility [8]. Haemorrhagic cystitis is a potentially fatal complication of CP, which is manifested by irritative voiding symptoms such as frequency, urgency and dysuria accompanied by microscopic or gross haematuria. The urotoxicity of CP is often dose-dependent and the incidence of haemorrhagic cystitis can vary ranging from 2 to 40%, which depends on total dose, the route of administration and duration of the treatment [9, 10]. In adults, the minimum cumulative oral dose of CP required for cystitis was reported as 100 g [11]. Patients receiving high doses of CP intravenously have been reported to be at the highest risk for the development of haemorrhagic cystitis, which mostly occurs within 48 hours of treatment. Late onset of haemorrhagic cystitis occurs rarely up to a month after the discontinuation of the drug. Concurrent use of other urotoxic chemotherapeutics and radiation therapy may increase the risk of haemorrhagic cystitis [10, 12]. Haemorrhagic cystitis arises from the direct effect of acrolein, which is a prominent urotoxic metabolite of CP on the bladder urothelium, leading to urothelial damage and ulceration. Acrolein is a highly reactive unsaturated aldehyde that is renally excreted into the urine and it accumulates in the bladder, which allows direct contact with the urothelium, consequently, damaging the bladder tissue by interacting with various mechanisms involved in oxidative stress and inflammatory response in the bladder [13, 14].

Ifosfamide (IFO) is an oxazaphosphorine derivative used for the treatment of paediatric, adolescent and young adult patients with a wide variety of malignancies, and it exhibits pharmacological effects via alkylating DNA, thus inhibiting DNA synthesis. Like CP, IFO is a prodrug that undergoes biotransformation mediated by CYP enzyme to yield phosphoramide mustard derivatives as active metabolites responsible for cytotoxic effects. IFO is also metabolised to acrolein, leading to haemorrhagic cystitis in the patients receiving IFO with an incidence rate of 20–40% [15, 16].

The clinical management of CP and IFO-induced haemorrhagic cystitis varies according to the severity of cases, thus therapeutic intervention should be selected depending on an individualised basis. Preventative measures remain the mainstay to reduce the risk of bladder inflammation, including hydration via intravenous or oral route and forced diuresis with furosemide if appreciated. Mild cases can be managed in an outpatient setting with hydration and anticholinergic drugs for lower urinary tract symptoms. Generally, intravenous hydration can provide sufficient treatment in cases without blood clots caused urinary tract obstruction [17, 18]. Sodium 2-mercaptoethane sulfonate (mesna) is an approved pharmacological tool used to prevent CP and IFO-induced haemorrhagic cystitis. Mesna acts as a thiol donor and thereby detoxifies the urotoxic metabolite acrolein, which significantly reduces the incidence of haemorrhagic cystitis induced by CP and IFO. Mesna is preferentially administrated intravenously in divided doses during the chemotherapy. Various protocols of administration for mesna have already been applied in clinical use [19, 20]. For the patients, given standard dose IFO (<2.5 g/m^2), a total daily dose of mesna is equal to 60% of the total daily dose of IFO, and mesna is administered as three bolus doses are given 15 minutes before, 4 and 8 hours after administration of each IFO dose. In case of oral administration of mesna, a total daily dose of mesna is the same as the total daily dose of IFO. Oral mesna should not be chosen as an initial dose and it can be applied after an intravenous bolus dose of mesna. [18, 21]. Mesna is especially recommended to use intravenously with forced saline diuresis for the patients given high-dose CP (50 mg/kg or 2 g/m^2). Continuous bladder irrigation may also be effective to avoid urinary exposures of the urothelium to acrolein and it is vital for the evacuation of all clots from the bladder in the treatment of intractable haematuria. Intravesical applications of formalin, alum 1% (potassium or ammonium aluminium sulphate), sodium hyaluronate, chondroitin sulphate, prostaglandin, and silver nitrate account for alternative options with varying degrees of efficacy [1, 4, 22]. Although hyperbaric oxygen is mainly preferred for radiation-induced cystitis, it may be effective in CP or IFO-induced haemorrhagic cystitis [1, 23]. Amifostine, dexamethasone, N-acetylcysteine, glutathione, pentosan polysulfate sodium, conjugated estrogens, recombinant factor VIIa and aminocaproic acid have also been shown to be beneficial.

Refractory severe cases with failure of pharmacological interventions should require surgical procedures including urinary diversion and cystectomy [4, 24]. Although many therapeutic approaches are currently available, they are not able to completely eliminate haemorrhagic cystitis. Thus, more efforts have been recently made for the discovery of novel options with improved efficacy in the treatment of CP and IFO-induced haemorrhagic cystitis [25–28].

3. Ketamine

Ketamine is primarily a non-competitive N-methyl-D-aspartate receptor antagonist that has been effectively used as a dissociative anaesthetic in humans and veterinary medicine since 1970 [29]. Ketamine has been also reported to exhibit pleiotropic effects such as sedative, antinociceptive, bronchodilatory, anticancer, antisuicidal, anti-inflammatory and immunomodulatory properties, which provides a wide range of potential therapeutic utility [30]. In recent years, ketamine has gained attention particularly due to its promising antidepressive effects in psychiatric research. In 2019, the *S*-enantiomer of ketamine in the form of an intranasal spray has recently been approved by the U.S. Food and Drug Administration (FDA) for the treatment of treatment-resistant depression [30, 31]. Apart from its therapeutic benefits, ketamine was reported to be one of the most frequently abused recreational drugs because of visual and auditory hallucinatory effects among drug addicts with its favourable properties such as rapid onset, short duration of action and low market price. Ketamine abuse is being dramatically increased worldwide, making its severe harms to individuals and society [30, 32].

Ketamine is chemically a phenylpiperidine derivate that possesses high lipophilicity, a plasma half-life of 2–4 h, relatively low protein binding and oral bioavailability. It can be applied via multiple routes including oral, intravenous, intramuscular, transdermal, subcutaneous, transdermal, intranasal, rectal and inhalation routes. However, abusers predominantly use ketamine intranasally because of the rapid onset of action and ease of administration. Ketamine is heavily metabolised by the hepatic CYP enzymes to produce an active metabolite called norketamine. Unchanged ketamine and its metabolites are excreted via urine [29, 30].

Chronic ketamine use or abuse has been reported to induce ulcerative cystitis with a broad spectrum of clinical symptoms ranging from polyuria, decreased bladder capacity, urgency, dysuria, nocturia, urinary incontinence and suprapubic pain to gross haematuria. Common histopathological features include the denudation of the urothelium, thickened bladder wall, lamina propria fibrosis and inflammation [33, 34]. The first case of ketamine-induced cystitis was described as an abuser in 2007, and approximately 30% of ketamine abusers have been reported to suffer from urinary problems. The severity of ketamine-associated lower urinary tract symptoms is significantly related to both the duration and the dosage of ketamine [1, 35]. Urological side effects of ketamine can develop when 2 g or more of ketamine is administered at least three times a week for 1 year. Therefore, therapeutic use of ketamine for anaesthesia at low doses (0.5–2 mg/kg) is considered to have no potential risk for cystitis. Urinary symptoms generally resolve after the discontinuation of ketamine, but in limited cases, they may last for up to 1 year after the cessation [36–38].

The pathogenesis of ketamine-induced cystitis is complicated and involves various mechanisms underlying the urothelial disruption, apoptosis, inflammation and fibrosis in the lamina propria; however, the precise mechanism remains largely unknown. The direct toxic effects of ketamine and norketamine on urothelium have been suggested to contribute to bladder damage [34]. There is currently no approved specific treatment for ketamine-induced cystitis. Currently, the cessation of ketamine is the only effective treatment and urinary symptoms can be improved by some symptomatic approaches including anticholinergic drugs, corticosteroids, intravesical injections of hyaluronic acid and botulinum toxin type A in the management of ketamine-induced cystitis [39].

4. Tiaprofenic acid

Tiaprofenic acid is a nonsteroidal anti-inflammatory drug (NSAID) with high potency as a cyclooxygenase inhibitor, which has been globally marketed for the treatment of rheumatic diseases and musculoskeletal disorders [40]. Tiaprofenic acid is rapidly and almost completely absorbed when orally administered. It has a high affinity for plasma proteins and a relatively short half-life (3 to 6 h). After extensively glucuronidated, nearly 60% of tiaprofenic acid is excreted via urine as glucuronide-conjugated metabolites [41].

Tiaprofenic acid-induced cystitis is well-documented and several cases have been published. Tiaprofenic acid was reported to cause usually late onset of urinary tract symptoms manifested by frequency, dysuria, urgency, suprapubic pain, haematuria and urinary incontinence with inflamed oedematous lamina propria as the main histological feature. According to case studies, urinary symptoms are observed to occur in 2 weeks and more than 2 years after the tiaprofenic acid has been started [42–44]. The aetiology is unclear; however, it can result from the direct toxic effect of tiaprofenic acid on the urothelium and a delayed hypersensitive immune response accompanied by the late onset of the symptoms [3]. It is recommended to stop tiaprofenic acid if urinary tract symptoms develop, which is able to resolve mild cases. More severe cases may require intravesical steroid instillation and surgical interventions such as cystoplasty and urinary diversion. Although the symptoms gradually improve within 6–14 weeks after the withdrawal of tiaprofenic acid, about 10% of cases can have residual symptoms due to persistent changes leading to bladder fibrosis. Tiaprofenic acid use should be avoided in patients with any history of urinary tract disorders [43, 44].

5. Mitomycin C

Mitomycin C is an alkylating chemotherapeutic drug that causes DNA damage by cross-linking DNA strands, thus inhibiting replication and transcription. Mitomycin C is indicated for various solid tumours including breast, gastric, bladder, pancreatic and non-small cell lung cancer [45]. Intravesical mitomycin C instillation is a standard care for non-muscle-invasive bladder cancer, which is highly effective in reducing the recurrence rate of superficial bladder cancer by up to 40%. It is recommended by the American Urological Association and European Association of Urology guidelines that mitomycin C should be applied intravesically at a dose of 40 mg following transurethral resection of bladder tumour [46, 47]. A common complication of intravesical mitomycin C is eosinophilic cystitis that is a rare form of allergic cystitis characterised by diffuse eosinophilic infiltration of lamina propria and muscularis with a spectrum of clinical presentations including dysuria, pelvic pain, haematuria, urinary urgency and urges incontinence [48, 49].

No approved treatment for mitomycin C-induced cystitis is currently available. It usually resolves spontaneously upon withdrawal of mitomycin C. Anticholinergics, antihistamines and alpha blockers can be used for 1–2 weeks in mild cases. If symptoms persist, prednisone (60 mg/day) should be prescribed for 2–4 weeks. Intravesical dimethyl sulfoxide and steroid injection can be applied when the symptoms do not completely improve or still persist due to initial treatments [49].

6. Penicillins

Penicillin is a pharmacological group of beta-lactam antibiotics that are widely used for various infectious diseases with favourable efficacy and safety profile. Penicillins are known to cause many kinds of side effects, however, haemorrhagic cystitis occurs on rare occasions [50].

Penicillin-induced cystitis is associated with deliberating urinary tract symptoms such as pyuria, dysuria, haematuria and frequency, along with predominantly eosinophilic infiltration of bladder. Penicillin G, methicillin, carbenicillin, ticarcillin and piperacillin have been implicated in the development of haemorrhagic cystitis. Urinary symptoms usually occur within 2 weeks after starting penicillin and disappear in few days following the withdrawal of penicillins. The exact mechanism of penicillin-induced cystitis still remains unclear, but it has been suggested that both an immunological mechanism resulting from penicillin-induced immune reaction and direct toxic effect of penicillins or metabolites are involved in bladder damage [4, 50, 51].

7. Immune checkpoint inhibitors

Immune checkpoint inhibitors (ICIs) have made a remarkable advance in the immunotherapy-based treatment of metastatic cancers since 2011 and they are being used increasingly worldwide [52]. ICIs are therapeutic humanised monoclonal antibodies that block receptors and ligands including cytotoxic T lymphocyte antigen-4, programmed death receptor-1 and programmed death ligand-1 involved in the inhibitory signals of T cells, thus allowing for robust activation of immune system and improved antitumor immune response. To date, seven ICIs have been approved for use in humans by FDA in the USA and several clinical trials are currently in progress [52, 53].

Despite that ICIs have provided considerable benefits for cancer patients, they are associated with diverse toxicities named immune-related adverse events (irAEs) resulting from the nonspecific overactivation of the immune system. irAEs represent a broad spectrum of dermatological, gastrointestinal and endocrine side effects and other organ system toxicities ranging from mild to life-threatening, which became a serious challenge for patients with the widespread use of ICIs [54]. Recently, few cases have described that ICIs including ipilimumab, atezolizumab, nivolumab, pembrolizumab and sintilimab are related to immune-related cystitis as an irAE [55–58]. ICIs-induced cystitis is generally manifested by irritative voiding symptoms and histological features of diffuse redness of bladder mucosa. Immune-related cystitis by ICIs can occur within 6 weeks but can also arise several years after the starting treatment [59]. Emerging evidence indicates that drug withdrawal and treatment with methylprednisolone or prednisolone are effective in the treatment of most cases, but infliximab can be used for steroid-refractory cases of immune-related cystitis [55]. Despite high efficacy of glucocorticoids, there are concerns about the use of glucocorticoids particularly as they are likely to affect negatively the therapeutic outcomes of ICIs due to immunosuppressive effects. Thus, unnecessary use of glucocorticoids should be avoided [58].

ICIs are associated with diverse irAEs of any grade that can develop in up to 30–60% of the patients of which 10–20% consist of severe cases. Among irAEs, immune-related cystitis is considered to be a rare complication of ICIs, therefore, the patients who are being treated with ICIs should be carefully monitored in order to detect early signs and recognise immune-related cystitis [53, 59].

8. Bacillus Calmette Guerin

Bacillus Calmette Guerin (BCG) is an attenuated strain of *Mycobacterium bovis*, which is primarily used for tuberculosis prevention as a vaccine. Intravesical instillation of BCG is the most effective therapy currently available for superficial bladder carcinoma after transurethral bladder cancer resection [60].

Intravesical BCG is commonly associated with various local and systemic complications ranging from mild to severe. BCG-related cystitis is the most frequent local complication occurring in up to 35% of patients and it is characterised by urination frequency, dysuria, bladder pain, transient haematuria with diffuse thickening of the bladder wall and oedematous mucosa [61, 62]. Cystitis induced by BCG has been shown to occur as a result of chemical or bacterial aetiology. Intravesical instillation of BCG leads to break down glycosaminoglycans layer that covers the urothelium of the bladder, which is the responsible for the initial step in the chemical pathological mechanism of BCG-related cystitis. Urinary symptoms usually develop within a few hours following BCG and generally resolve within 48 hours, demonstrating a hypersensitivity reaction to BCG antigens in the pathogenesis of BCG-related cystitis [1, 61, 62]. Bacterial cystitis due to *M. bovis* may occur and persist long-term after intravesical BCG administration. Antimycobacterial agents, glucocorticoids and hyperbaric oxygen are useful to improve BCG-related cystitis, in addition, NSAIDs and anticholinergic agents may be proposed to alleviate the symptoms of BCG-related cystitis [63–65].

9. Miscellaneous drugs

CP and IFO are alkylating agents that are well-known to be causative drugs for haemorrhagic cystitis. It has been demonstrated that other alkylating agents such as busulfan, thiotepa, temozolomide and dacarbazine can also potentially induce cystitis that could be clinically managed with the discontinuation of the drug and continuous bladder irrigation [66–69]. Chemotherapeutic agents are also employed for intravesical therapy to treat bladder cancer due to its lower risk potential for recurrence and adverse effects. Intravesical administration of doxorubicin, epirubicin, valrubicin, ethoglucid, cisplatin and mitoxantrone has been reported to cause bladder damage [2, 70]. Especially, gross haematuria can occur in 20% of patients when doxorubicin is combined with mitomycin C, leading to discontinuation of the therapy [71]. On rare occasions, taxanes are also associated with haemorrhagic cystitis. Cabazitaxel, docetaxel, solvent-based and albumin-bound paclitaxel have been reported to induce haemorrhagic cystitis that resolved after the drug withdrawal or bladder irrigation [72–74]. The patients treated with cabazitaxel were previously exposed to pelvic radiation in most cases of cystitis, suggesting that radiation recall syndrome induced by cabazitaxel may be implicated in cabazitaxel-related cystitis [74]. However, cabazitaxel-related haemorrhagic cystitis was even seen in a patient without a history of radiation therapy [75]. Gefitinib is an oral epidermal growth factor receptor tyrosine kinase (EGFR) inhibitor that has been widely used as a first-line treatment of advanced non-small cell lung cancer with proven efficacy after standard chemotherapy [76]. Gefitinib-related cystitis has been rarely reported and the precise mechanism is yet to be defined. But it was speculated that the EGFR signalling pathway affected by gefitinib could mediate the alterations in the bladder [77].

NSAIDs are one of the most widely used drugs to treat a broad range of diseases due to their antipyretic, analgesic and anti-inflammatory properties. Despite being commonly available without a prescription, NSAIDs have potential safety concerns because of numerous adverse effects in long-term use. Tiaprofenic acid seems to have a higher risk of cystitis, however, other NSAIDs like indomethacin, diclofenac, ketoprofen, naproxen and piroxicam have been reported to be associated with cystitis [3, 78].

Statins are the inhibitors of the hydroxymethylglutaryl-CoA reductase enzyme that catalyses the crucial step of cholesterol biosynthesis and they are highly effective drugs in hyperlipidaemia. Statin use was found to be significantly associated with interstitial cystitis [79]. Moreover, haemorrhagic cystitis was reported in a patient receiving atorvastatin in the 2nd week of the treatment and haematuria disappeared within 1 week after the withdrawal of atorvastatin [80]. The mechanisms of statin-related cystitis are largely unclarified; however, statins have been shown to induce chronic inflammation in the urothelium [79].

Emphysematous cystitis is a relatively rare form of complicated urinary tract infection commonly seen in elderly females with diabetes, which is characterised by gas within the bladder wall and lumen due to gas-producing bacteria [81]. It has been reported that sodium-glucose cotransporter-2 inhibitors such as empagliflozin may increase the risk for emphysematous cystitis in diabetic patients [82].

Acetylsalicylic acid and dabigatran have been related to haemorrhagic cystitis with unknown aetiology [83, 84]. In addition, it should be noticed that anticoagulants and antiplatelet drugs can exacerbate bleeding in the patients' receiving drugs that induce haemorrhagic cystitis [85].

Other drugs have been associated with cystitis include allopurinol, danazol, methaqualone, methenamine mandelate, tacrolimus and tranilast [86–90].

10. Conclusions

Cystitis is considered to be unusual for being a side effect of drugs, except with some chemotherapeutics. Therefore, drug-related cystitis is likely to be a less recognised and underestimated condition that leads to impaired quality of patients' life, discontinuation of medication and non-compliance. To date, several drugs have been reported to induce cystitis. Although CP or IFO-induced cystitis can be treated with well-established pharmacological approaches, there is no currently approved treatment for another drugs-related cystitis. However, discontinuation of suspected drugs and glucocorticoids have been proven to be effective in most cases. Infliximab may also be indicated for steroid-resistant cystitis. Moreover, surgical interventions should be employed in severe cases. Patients taking drugs who suffer from urinary problems should be advised to seek prompt medical attention. Physicians should be also aware of the potential association between drug use and cystitis in patients with clinical presentation of cystitis.

Author details

Seçkin Engin
Faculty of Pharmacy, Department of Pharmacology, Karadeniz Technical University, Trabzon, Türkiye

*Address all correspondence to: seckinengin@ktu.edu.tr

References

[1] Petca RC, Popescu RI, Toma C, Dumitrascu MC, Petca A, Sandru F, et al. Chemical hemorrhagic cystitis: Diagnostic and therapeutic pitfalls (review). Experimental and Therapeutic Medicine. 2021;**21**(6):624. DOI: 10.3892/etm.2021.10056

[2] Drake MJ, Nixon PM, Crew JP. Drug-induced bladder and urinary disorders. Incidence, prevention and management. Drug Safety. 1998;**19**(1):45-55. DOI: 10.2165/00002018-199819010-00004

[3] Bramble FJ, Morley R. Drug-induced cystitis: The need for vigilance. British Journal of Urology. 1997;**79**(1):3-7. DOI: 10.1046/j.1464-410x.1997.02761.x

[4] Manikandan R, Kumar S, Dorairajan LN. Hemorrhagic cystitis: A challenge to the urologist. Indian Journal of Urology. 2010;**26**(2):159-166. DOI: 10.4103/0970-1591.65380

[5] Yuksel OH, Urkmez A, Erdogru T, Verit A. The role of steroid treatment in intractable cystitis glandularis: A case report and literature review. Canadian Urological Association Journal. 2015;**9**(5-6):E306-E309. DOI: 10.5489/cuaj.2636

[6] Giraud B, Hebert G, Deroussent A, Veal GJ, Vassal G, Paci A. Oxazaphosphorines: New therapeutic strategies for an old class of drugs. Expert Opinion on Drug Metabolism & Toxicology. 2010;**6**(8):919-938. DOI: 10.1517/17425255.2010.487861

[7] Emadi A, Jones RJ, Brodsky RA. Cyclophosphamide and cancer: Golden anniversary. Nature Reviews. Clinical Oncology. 2009;**6**(11):638-647. DOI: 10.1038/nrclinonc.2009

[8] Fraiser LH, Kanekal S, Kehrer JP. Cyclophosphamide toxicity. Characterising and avoiding the problem. Drugs. 1991;**42**(5):781-795. DOI: 10.2165/00003495-199142050-00005

[9] Levine LA, Richie JP. Urological complications of cyclophosphamide. The Journal of Urology. 1989;**141**(5):1063-1069. DOI: 10.1016/s0022-5347(17)41173-6

[10] Manikandan R, Kumar S, Dorairajan LN. Hemorrhagic cystitis: A challenge to the urologist. Indian Journal of Urology. 2010;**26**(2):159-166. DOI: 10.4103/0970-1591.65380

[11] Spiers AS, Chikkappa G, Wilbur HJ. Hemorrhagic cystitis after low-dose cyclophosphamide. Lancet. 1983;**1**(8335):1213-1214. DOI: 10.1016/s0140-6736(83)92484-4

[12] Doshi BR, Sajjan VV, Manjunathswamy BS. Managing a side effect: Cyclophosphamide-induced hemorrhagic cystitis. Indian Journal of Drugs Dermatology. 2019;**5**:66-71. DOI: 10.4103/ijdd.ijdd_31_19

[13] Korkmaz A, Topal T, Oter S. Pathophysiological aspects of cyclophosphamide and ifosfamide induced hemorrhagic cystitis; implication of reactive oxygen and nitrogen species as well as PARP activation. Cell Biology and Toxicology. 2007;**23**(5):303-312. DOI: 10.1007/s10565-006-0078-0

[14] Cox PJ. Cyclophosphamide cystitis-identification of acrolein as the causative agent. Biochem Pharmacol. 1979;**28**(13):2045-9. DOI: 10.1016/0006-2952(79)90222-3

[15] Matz EL, Hsieh MH. Review of advances in Uroprotective agents for cyclophosphamide- and Ifosfamide-induced hemorrhagic cystitis. Urology. 2017;**100**:16-19. DOI: 10.1016/j.urology.2016.07.030

[16] Brade WP, Herdrich K, Varini M. Ifosfamide--pharmacology, safety and therapeutic potential. Cancer Treatment Reviews. 1985;**12**(1):1-47. DOI: 10.1016/0305-7372(85)90011-8

[17] Johnston D, Schurtz E, Tourville E, Jones T, Boemer A, Giel D. Risk factors associated with severity and outcomes in pediatric patients with hemorrhagic cystitis. The Journal of Urology. 2016;**195**(4 Pt 2):1312-1317. DOI: 10.1016/j.juro.2015.11.035

[18] Hensley ML, Hagerty KL, Kewalramani T, Green DM, Meropol NJ, Wasserman TH, et al. American Society of Clinical Oncology 2008 clinical practice guideline update: Use of chemotherapy and radiation therapy protectants. Journal of Clinical Oncology. 2009;**27**(1):127-145. DOI: 10.1200/JCO.2008.17.2627

[19] West NJ. Prevention and treatment of hemorrhagic cystitis. Pharmacotherapy. 1997;**17**(4):696-706

[20] Mukhtar S, Woodhouse C. The management of cyclophosphamide-induced haematuria. BJU International. 2010;**105**(7):908-912. DOI: 10.1111/j.1464-410X.2009.09132

[21] Katz A, Epelman S, Anelli A, Gorender EF, Cruz SM, Oliveira RM, et al. A prospective randomized evaluation of three schedules of mesna administration in patients receiving an ifosfamide-containing chemotherapy regimen: Sustained efficiency and simplified administration. Journal of Cancer Research and Clinical Oncology. 1995;**121**(2):128-131. DOI: 10.1007/BF01202226

[22] Gonella S, di Pasquale T, Palese A. Preventive measures for cyclophosphamide-related hemorrhagic cystitis in blood and bone marrow transplantation: An Italian multicenter retrospective study. Clinical Journal of Oncology Nursing. 2015;**19**(1):E8-E14. DOI: 10.1188/15.CJON.E8-E14

[23] Weiss JP, Boland FP, Mori H, Gallagher M, Brereton H, Preate DL, et al. Treatment of radiation-induced cystitis with hyperbaric oxygen. The Journal of Urology. 1985;**134**(2):352-354. DOI: 10.1016/s0022-5347(17)47166-7

[24] D'Amico MJ, Foss H, Uhr A, Rudnick B, Kloniecke E, Gomella LG. Hemorrhagic cystitis: A review of the literature and treatment options. The Canadian Journal of Urology. 2022;**29**(5):11276-11283

[25] Engin S, Barut EN, Soysal AC, Keskin O, Kerimoglu G, Kadioglu M, et al. Double benefit of metformin treatment: Improved bladder function in cyclophosphamide-induced cystitis and enhanced cytotoxicity in cancer cells. Naunyn-Schmiedeberg's Archives of Pharmacology. 2021;**394**(6):1167-1175. DOI: 10.1007/s00210-021-02055-9

[26] Engin S, Barut EN, Yaşar YK, Soysal AÇ, Arıcı T, Kerimoğlu G, et al. Trimetazidine attenuates cyclophosphamide-induced cystitis by inhibiting TLR4-mediated NFκB signaling in mice. Life Sciences. 2022;**301**:120590. DOI: 10.1016/j.lfs.2022.120590

[27] Almeida de Oliveira LS, de Moura Bandeira SR, Gomes Gonçalves RL, Pereira de Sousa Neto B, Carvalho de Rezende D, Dos Reis-Filho AC, et al. The isopropyl Gallate counteracts cyclophosphamide-induced

hemorrhagic cystitis in mice. Biology (Basel). 2022;**11**(5):728. DOI: 10.3390/biology11050728

[28] Gonçalves RLG, Cunha FVM, Sousa-Neto BPS, Oliveira LSA, Lopes ME, Rezende DC, et al. α-Phellandrene attenuates tissular damage, oxidative stress, and TNF-α levels on acute model ifosfamide-induced hemorrhagic cystitis in mice. Naunyn-Schmiedeberg's Archives of Pharmacology. 2020;**393**(10):1835-1848. DOI: 10.1007/s00210-020-01869-3

[29] Zanos P, Moaddel R, Morris PJ, Riggs LM, Highland JN, Georgiou P, et al. Ketamine and ketamine metabolite pharmacology: Insights into therapeutic mechanisms. Pharmacological Reviews. 2018;**70**(3):621-660. DOI: 10.1124/pr.117.015198

[30] Nowacka A, Borczyk M. Ketamine applications beyond anesthesia - a literature review. European Journal of Pharmacology. 2019;**860**:172547. DOI: 10.1016/j.ejphar.2019.172547

[31] Iqbal SZ, Mathew SJ. Ketamine for depression clinical issues. Advances in Pharmacology. 2020;**89**:131-162. DOI: 10.1016/bs.apha.2020.02.005

[32] Bokor G, Anderson PD. Ketamine: An update on its abuse. Journal of Pharmacy Practice. 2014;**27**(6):582-586. DOI: 10.1177/0897190014525754

[33] Tsai TH, Cha TL, Lin CM, Tsao CW, Tang SH, Chuang FP, et al. Ketamine-associated bladder dysfunction. International Journal of Urology. 2009;**16**(10):826-829. DOI: 10.1111/j.1442-2042.2009.02361.x

[34] Xie X, Liang J, Huang R, Luo C, Yang J, Xing H, et al. Molecular pathways underlying tissue injuries in the bladder with ketamine cystitis. The FASEB Journal. 2021;**35**(7):e21703. DOI: 10.1096/fj.202100437

[35] Sultana S, Berger G, Cox A, Kelly MEM, Lehmann C. Rodent models of ketamine-induced cystitis. Neurourology and Urodynamics. 2021;**40**(7):1704-1719. DOI: 10.1002/nau.24763

[36] Castellani D, Pirola GM, Gubbiotti M, Rubilotta E, Gudaru K, Gregori A, et al. What urologists need to know about ketamine-induced uropathy: A systematic review. Neurourology and Urodynamics. 2020;**39**(4):1049-1062

[37] Lai Y, Wu S, Ni L, Chen Z, Li X, Yang S, et al. Ketamine-associated urinary tract dysfunction: An underrecognized clinical entity. Urologia Internationalis. 2012;**89**(1):93-96. DOI: 10.1159/000338098

[38] Shung-Lai Leung J, Ma W-K. Urological effects of ketamine abuse. In: Biomarkers and Bioanalysis Overview. London, UK: IntechOpen; 2021. DOI: 10.5772/intechopen.91283

[39] Jhang JF, Hsu YH, Kuo HC. Possible pathophysiology of ketamine-related cystitis and associated treatment strategies. International Journal of Urology. 2015;**22**(9):816-825. DOI: 10.1111/iju.12841

[40] Sorkin EM, Brogden RN, Tiaprofenic acid. A review of its pharmacological properties and therapeutic efficacy in rheumatic diseases and pain states. Drugs. 1985;**29**(3):208-235. DOI: 10.2165/00003495-198529030-00002

[41] Davies NM. Clinical pharmacokinetics of tiaprofenic acid and its enantiomers. Clinical Pharmacokinetics. 1996;**31**(5):331-347. DOI: 10.2165/00003088-199631050-00002

[42] Andreassen KH, Eldrup J, Hansen RI, Oster S. Tiaprofenic acid-induced cystitis--three cases and a literature review. Scandinavian Journal of Urology and Nephrology. 1999;**33**(6):408-410. DOI: 10.1080/003655999750017095

[43] Bateman DN. Tiaprofenic acid and cystitis. BMJ. 1994;**309**(6954):552-553. DOI: 10.1136/bmj.309.6954.552

[44] Henley MJ, Harriss D, Bishop MC. Cystitis associated with tiaprofenic acid: A survey of British and Irish urologists. British Journal of Urology. 1997;**79**(4):585-587. DOI: 10.1046/j.1464-410x.1997.00125.x

[45] Bradner WT. Mitomycin C: a clinical update. Cancer Treatment Reviews. 2001;**27**(1):35-50. DOI: 10.1053/ctrv.2000.0202

[46] Sylvester RJ, Oosterlinck W, van der Meijden AP. A single immediate postoperative instillation of chemotherapy decreases the risk of recurrence in patients with stage Ta T1 bladder cancer: A meta-analysis of published results of randomized clinical trials. The Journal of Urology. 2004;**171**(6 Pt 1):2186-2190, quiz 2435. DOI: 10.1097/01.ju.0000125486.92260.b2

[47] Babjuk M, Burger M, Zigeuner R, Shariat SF, van Rhijn BW, Compérat E, et al. EAU guidelines on non-muscle-invasive urothelial carcinoma of the bladder: Update 2013. European Urology. 2013;**64**(4):639-653. DOI: 10.1016/j.eururo.2013.06.003

[48] Ulker V, Apaydin E, Gürsan A, Ozyurt C, Kandiloğlu G. Eosinophilic cystitis induced by mitomycin-C. International Urology and Nephrology. 1996;**28**(6):755-759. DOI: 10.1007/BF02550723

[49] Luckenbaugh AN, Marks RM, Miller DC, Weizer AZ, Stoffel JT, Montgomery JS. A management algorithm for Mitomycin C induced cystitis. Bladder Cancer. 2017;**3**(2):133-138. DOI: 10.3233/BLC-160089

[50] Kim MK, Kang CK, Kim MJ, Jun KI, Lee YK, Jeong SJ, et al. Penicillin G-induced hemorrhagic cystitis: A case and review of the literature. The Korean Journal of Internal Medicine. 2013;**28**(6):743-745. DOI: 10.3904/kjim.2013.28.6.743

[51] Tsakiri A, Balslev I, Klarskov P. Eosinophilic cystitis induced by penicillin. International Urology and Nephrology. 2004;**36**(2):159-161. DOI: 10.1023/b:urol.0000034663.53795.25

[52] Chhabra N, Kennedy J. A review of cancer immunotherapy toxicity: Immune checkpoint inhibitors. Journal of Medical Toxicology. 2021;**17**(4):411-424. DOI: 10.1007/s13181-021-00833-8

[53] Bagchi S, Yuan R, Engleman EG. Immune checkpoint inhibitors for the treatment of cancer: Clinical impact and mechanisms of response and resistance. Annual Review of Pathology. 2021;**16**:223-249. DOI: 10.1146/annurev-pathol-042020-042741

[54] Johnson DB, Nebhan CA, Moslehi JJ, Balko JM. Immune-checkpoint inhibitors: Long-term implications of toxicity. Nature Reviews. Clinical Oncology. 2022;**19**(4):254-267. DOI: 10.1038/s41571-022-00600-w

[55] Fukunaga H, Sumii K, Kawamura S, Okuno M, Taguchi I, Kawabata G. A case of steroid-resistant cystitis as an immune-related adverse event during treatment with nivolumab for lung cancer, which was successfully treated with infliximab. IJU Case Report.

2022;**5**(6):521-523. DOI: 10.1002/iju5.12532

[56] Tu L, Ye Y, Tang X, Liang Z, You Q, Zhou J, et al. Case report: A case of Sintilimab-induced cystitis/Ureteritis and review of Sintilimab-related adverse events. Frontiers in Oncology. 2021;**11**:757069. DOI: 10.3389/fonc.2021.757069

[57] He X, Tu R, Zeng S, He Z, Liu S, Fang Y. Non-bacterial cystitis secondary to pembrolizumab: A case report and review of the literature. Current Problems in Cancer. 2022;**46**(4):100863. DOI: 10.1016/j.currproblcancer.2022.100863

[58] Obayashi A, Hamada-Nishimoto M, Fujimoto Y, Yoshimoto Y, Takahara S. Non-bacterial cystitis with increased expression of programmed cell death ligand 1 in the Urothelium: An unusual immune-related adverse event after Atezolizumab Administration for Metastatic Breast Cancer. Cureus. 2022;**14**(5):e25486. DOI: 10.7759/cureus.25486

[59] Zhu L, Wang Z, Stebbing J, Wang Z, Peng L. Immunotherapy-related cystitis: Case report and review of the literature. Oncotargets and Therapy. 2021;**14**:4321-4328. DOI: 10.2147/OTT.S321965

[60] Han J, Gu X, Li Y, Wu Q. Mechanisms of BCG in the treatment of bladder cancer-current understanding and the prospect. Biomedicine & Pharmacotherapy. 2020;**129**:110393. DOI: 10.1016/j.biopha.2020.110393

[61] Decaestecker K, Oosterlinck W. Managing the adverse events of intravesical bacillus Calmette-Guérin therapy. Research and Reports in Urology. 2015;7:157-163. DOI: 10.2147/RRU.S63448

[62] Hidoussi A, Slama A, Jaidane M, Zakhama W, Youssef A, Ben Sorba N, et al. Eosinophilic cystitis induced by bacillus Calmette-Guerin (BCG) intravesical instillation. Urology. 2007;**70**(3):591.e9-591.10. DOI: 10.1016/j.urology.2007.07.032

[63] Ströck V, Dotevall L, Sandberg T, Gustafsson CK, Holmäng S. Late bacille Calmette-Guérin infection with a large focal urinary bladder ulceration as a complication of bladder cancer treatment. BJU International. 2011;**107**(10):1592-1597. DOI: 10.1111/j.1464-410X.2010.09923.x

[64] Palou J, Rodríguez-Villamil L, Andreu-Crespo A, Salvador-Bayarri J, Vicente-Rodríguez J. Intravesical treatment of severe bacillus Calmette-Guerin cystitis. International Urology and Nephrology. 2001;**33**(3):485-489. DOI: 10.1023/a:1019507104741

[65] Markovitz GH. Two cases of bacillus Calmette-Guérin cystitis treated with hyperbaric oxygen. Undersea & Hyperbaric Medicine. 2022;**49**(2):191-195

[66] Millard RJ. Busulfan-induced hemorrhagic cystitis. Urology. 1981;**18**(2):143-144. DOI: 10.1016/0090-4295(81)90424-6

[67] Choe JM, Kirkemo AK, Sirls LT. Intravesical thiotepa-induced eosinophilic cystitis. Urology. 1995;**46**(5):729-731. DOI: 10.1016/S0090-4295(99)80312-4

[68] Islam R, Isaacson BJ, Zickerman PM, Ratanawong C, Tipping SJ. Hemorrhagic cystitis as an unexpected adverse reaction to temozolomide: Case report. American Journal of Clinical Oncology. 2002;**25**(5):513-514. DOI: 10.1097/00000421-200210000-00018

[69] Mohammadianpanah M, Shirazi M, Mosalaei A, Omidvari S, Ahmadloo N. Hemorrhagic cystitis in a patient receiving conventional doses of dacarbazine for metastatic malignant melanoma: Case report and review of the literature. Clinical Therapeutics. 2007;**29**(6):1161-1165. DOI: 10.1016/j.clinthera.2007.06.004

[70] Raspollini MR, Lopez-Beltran A. Cystitis after chemotherapy. In: Raspollini MR, Lopez-Beltran A, editors. Uropathology. Encyclopedia of Pathology. Cham: Springer; 2020. DOI: 10.1007/978-3-030-41894-6_3740

[71] Fukui I, Sekine H, Kihara K, Yamada T, Takeuchi S, Yokokawa M, et al. Intravesical combination chemotherapy with mitomycin C and doxorubicin for carcinoma in situ of the bladder. The Journal of Urology. 1989;**141**(3):531-534. DOI: 10.1016/s0022-5347(17)40882-2

[72] Ichioka E, Iguchi-Manaka A, Oikawa T, Sawa A, Okazaki M, Saito T, et al. A case of hemorrhagic cystitis caused by nab-paclitaxel. International Cancer Conference Journal. 2016;**5**(4):187-191. DOI: 10.1007/s13691-016-0255-9

[73] Ntekim AI, Ajekigbe A. Hemorrhagic cystitis in a patient receiving docetaxel for prostate cancer. Clinical Medicine Insights: Oncology. 2010;**4**:11-13. DOI: 10.4137/cmo.s4477

[74] Grellety T, Houédé N, Hoepffner JL, Rivière J, Mérino C, Lieutenant V, et al. Hemorrhagic cystitis in patients treated with cabazitaxel: A radiation recall syndrome? Annals of Oncology. 2014;**25**(6):1248-1249. DOI: 10.1093/annonc/mdu132

[75] Kosaka T, Oya M. Hemorrhagic cystitis in a patient without a past history of radiation therapy who was treated with cabazitaxel for CRPC. Annals of Oncology. 2015;**26**(11):2355-2356. DOI: 10.1093/annonc/mdv362

[76] Yang Z, Hackshaw A, Feng Q, Fu X, Zhang Y, Mao C, et al. Comparison of gefitinib, erlotinib and afatinib in non-small cell lung cancer: A meta-analysis. International Journal of Cancer. 2017;**140**(12):2805-2819. DOI: 10.1002/ijc.30691

[77] Bai X, Cheng J, Zhao L, Cheng M. Gefitinib-induced hemorrhagic cystitis and inflammatory contracted bladder in a patient with advanced lung adenocarcinoma harboring compound epidermal growth factor receptor G719S and S768I missense mutations: A case report. Annals of Translational Medicine. 2022;**10**(14):809. DOI: 10.21037/atm-22-3233

[78] Ghose K. Cystitis and nonsteroidal antiinflammatory drugs: An incidental association or an adverse effect? The New Zealand Medical Journal. 1993;**106**(968):501-503

[79] Huang CY, Chung SD, Kao LT, Lin HC, Wang LH. Statin use is associated with bladder pain syndrome/interstitial cystitis: A population-based case-control study. Urologia Internationalis. 2015;**95**(2):227-232. DOI: 10.1159/000431185

[80] Martinez-Suarez HJ, Wang R, Faerber GJ. Atorvastatin-induced hemorrhagic cystitis: A case report. Urology. 2009;**73**(3):681.e5-681.e6. DOI: 10.1016/j.urology.2008.03.027

[81] Amano M, Shimizu T. Emphysematous cystitis: A review of the literature. Internal Medicine. 2014;**53**(2):79-82. DOI: 10.2169/internalmedicine.53.1121

[82] Brock GM, Lane SM, Roosevelt TS. Emphysematous cystitis and urinary

retention in a male patient with diabetes mellitus type 2 treated with Empagliflozin. AACE Clinical Case Reports. 2022;**8**(4):163-165. DOI: 10.1016/j.aace.2022.04.002

[83] Avidor Y, Nadu A, Matzkin H. Clinical significance of gross hematuria and its evaluation in patients receiving anticoagulant and aspirin treatment. Urology. 2000;**55**(1):22-24. DOI: 10.1016/s0090-4295(99)00388-x

[84] Otteno H, Smith E, Huffaker RK. Dabigatran induced hemorrhagic cystitis in a patient with painful bladder syndrome. Case Reports in Urology. 2014;**2014**:871481. DOI: 10.1155/2014/871481

[85] Russo P. Urologic emergencies in the cancer patient. Seminars in Oncology. 2000;**27**(3):284-298

[86] Bramble FJ, Morley R. Cystitis associated with allopurinol. British Journal of Urology. 1997;**79**(5):817. DOI: 10.1046/j.1464-410x.1997.00216.x

[87] Andriole GL, Brickman C, Lack EE, et al. Danazol-induced cystitis: An undescribed source of hematuria in patients with hereditary angioneurotic edema. The Journal of Urology. 1986;**135**(1):44-46. DOI: 10.1016/s0022-5347(17)45509-1

[88] Goldfarb M, Finelli R. Necrotizing cystitis. Secondary to "bootleg" methaqualone. Urology. 1974;**3**(1):54-55. DOI: 10.1016/s0090-4295(74)80061-0

[89] Ross RR Jr, Conway GF. Hemorrhagic cystitis following accidental overdose of methenamine mandelate. American Journal of Diseases of Children. 1970;**119**(1):86-87. DOI: 10.1001/archpedi.1970.02100050088021

[90] Min IS, Ju Y, Kim HY, Choi YJ, Lee WS, Yoo WH. Hemorrhagic cystitis with Giant cells in rheumatoid arthritis treating with tacrolimus. Journal of Rheumatic Diseases. 2014;**21**:336-339. DOI: 10.4078/jrd.2014.21.6.336